VACCINATING AMERICA

THE INSIDE STORY BEHIND THE RACE TO SAVE LIVES AND END A PANDEMIC

For access to digital chapters,
visit the APHA Press bookstore (www.apha.org).

VACCINATING AMERICA

THE INSIDE STORY BEHIND THE RACE
TO SAVE LIVES AND END A PANDEMIC

MICHAEL FRASER, PhD, MS
BRENT EWIG, MHS

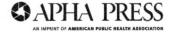
APHA PRESS
AN IMPRINT OF AMERICAN PUBLIC HEALTH ASSOCIATION

American Public Health Association
800 I Street, NW
Washington, DC 20001-3710
www.apha.org

Georges C. Benjamin, MD, MACP, Executive Director

Printed and bound in the United States of America
Book Production Editor: Maya Ribault
Typesetter: KnowledgeWorks Global, Ltd.
Cover Design: Alan Giarcanella
Printing and Binding: Sheridan Books

Library of Congress Cataloging-in-Publication Data

Names: Fraser, Michael R., author. | Ewig, Brent, author.
Title: Vaccinating America : the inside story behind the race to save lives
   and end a pandemic / Michael Fraser, PhD, Brent Ewig, MHS.
Description: Washington, DC : American Public Health Association, [2022] |
   Includes bibliographical references and index. | Summary: "The rapid
   development of vaccines against COVID is an astounding achievement. This
   book tells the story of how this unprecedented and historic vaccine
   distribution campaign took place in America"-- Provided by publisher.
Identifiers: LCCN 2022041698 (print) | LCCN 2022041699 (ebook) | ISBN
   9780875533322 (paperback) | ISBN 9780875533339 (adobe pdf)
Subjects: LCSH: COVID-19 (Disease)--Vaccination--United States. |
   Vaccines--Development--United States. | Public health
   administration--United States. | Vaccination--Social aspects--United
   States. | Vaccine hesitancy--United States.
Classification: LCC RA644.C67 F737 2022 (print) | LCC RA644.C67 (ebook) |
   DDC 362.1962/4144--dc23/eng/20221017
LC record available at https://lccn.loc.gov/2022041698
LC ebook record available at https://lccn.loc.gov/2022041699

To the countless public servants, public health leaders, health professionals, and private-sector partners who together ran the race to vaccinate America. We salute you for your service and appreciate the sacrifices you make daily to keep America healthy.

Contents

Preface

We are moved by sensational images of heroes who leap into action as calamity unfolds before them. But the long, pedestrian slog of prevention is thankless. That is because prevention is nameless and abstract, while a hero's actions are grounded in an easy-to-understand narrative.[1]

–Nassim Nicholas Taleb

The rapid development of vaccines against COVID is an astounding achievement. Only 339 days lapsed between the release of the SARS-CoV-2 genetic code and a nurse named Sandra Lindsay receiving the first COVID vaccine outside of a clinical trial in New York City on December 14, 2020.[2] What happened in the 365 days following that first shot is perhaps even more astounding. The US government delivered close to 600 million doses of COVID vaccine in that short time, with health officials, pharmacists, and other health care providers fully vaccinating over 60% of the population and providing protection against serious illness and death to over 200 million Americans.[3]

This book tells the story of how this unprecedented and historic vaccine distribution campaign took place. The endeavor was the most complicated vaccination campaign in American history, but the results have been extraordinary. The Commonwealth Fund estimates that through March 2022 the American vaccination campaign has saved over 2.2 million lives, prevented over 17 million hospitalizations, and avoided nearly $900 billion in health care costs.[4] While challenges to vaccinating all Americans remain, by most measures the race to vaccinate America has been a triumph.

When we began this project, our intent was to describe the unprecedented vaccination effort, successful despite its many technical and political challenges. When we began writing in the summer of 2021, vaccine demand was high, access to free vaccines had expanded dramatically, and COVID cases and deaths were falling fast. Americans everywhere were hopeful that the worst of the pandemic was behind us. But as summer progressed, the combination of entrenched vaccine hesitancy and the emergence of a more infectious COVID variant, Delta, caused additional surges of hospitalizations and deaths. Many of these hospitalizations and deaths were among individuals who had chosen not to get vaccinated.

As of this writing, tens of millions of Americans have declined to be vaccinated. Tragically, 400,000 citizens have died since free, effective, lifesaving vaccines became widely available.[5] This preventable morbidity and mortality also clearly points to missed opportunities and the deeper failings of America's public health and health care systems. As such, we consider the factors contributing to the campaign's success, as well as those that inhibited or are still inhibiting progress, with an eye toward improvements.

UNPRECEDENTED. HISTORIC. ONCE IN A LIFETIME.

Unprecedented. Historic. Once in a lifetime. These words are used to describe the COVID pandemic that to date has killed over six million worldwide and more than one million people in the United States. These words can also be used to describe the political and public health response to the emerging pathogen. Too often, public health and broader governmental achievements go unnoticed and underappreciated. Our intent also is to hold up the COVID vaccination campaign as one of the greatest achievements of modern American government, possible only through the leadership of many and the dedication and commitment of all involved.

But never has the US public health system faced such national scrutiny and criticism for its valiant attempts to contain and control an emerging infection. Since the onset of the COVID pandemic, the world experienced devastating loss of life from the SARS-CoV-2 virus, societies shut down, and travel ceased as part of global efforts to prevent transmission of the virus. The quick spread of the SARS-CoV-2 virus and accompanying illness and death earned a place in history as a once-in-100-years plague akin to and now exceeding the pandemic flu of 1918.[6] The economy was losing billions of dollars in addition to millions of jobs, businesses, and livelihoods.

In response, the US Congress appropriated over $5 trillion to mitigate the health and economic effects of the virus.[7] Of this total, approximately $482 billion was dedicated to bolstering federal, state, and local governmental public health responses to the emerging pathogen, to caring for the sick, and to taking steps to mitigate and contain it.[8] Of this, approximately $40 billion was dedicated to the research, manufacture, purchase, distribution, and administration of safe and effective COVID vaccines. The return on investment for this $40 billion should go down in history as one of the most effective public investments ever.

In a world connected by social media and a 24-hour news cycle, the often-invisible work of public health professionals was made plain and clear in daily headlines resulting in both praise of public health officials and rage against science-based efforts to prevent infection. After safe, effective vaccines were quickly developed to prevent illness and infection, the politicization of the public health response and distrust of public health guidance and recommendations remained high. This resulted in a significant portion of Americans choosing to not get vaccinated, leaving themselves unprotected, endangering those who cannot be vaccinated either because of age or medical conditions, increasing the chances that a vaccine-resistant variant emerges, potentially extending the pandemic, and stymying public health officials' efforts to reopen businesses and schools and to return to "normal."

Many who initially chose not to be vaccinated had rational reasons. Some were concerned about how fast the vaccine was developed and wanted to wait to see if it was safe before they got vaccinated. Many people from communities of color were concerned about past mistreatment and contemporary discrimination and racism in the medical establishment and lacked trust in public health authorities. But perhaps most unpredictably, political party affiliation became one of the strongest predictors of vaccination status. Anti-vaccination and anti-science activists leveraged COVID as a chance to spread disinformation and sow conspiracies and distrust. As a result, health authorities have had to confront vaccine hesitancy as never before. Confronting this hesitancy is a critical challenge for the future of our COVID response, as well as for any public health campaign in the future.

IN THE ARENA

We witnessed and experienced the pandemic and the Herculean effort to vaccinate America from unique perspectives. As chief executive officer of the Association of State and Territorial Health Officials, Michael Fraser had a front row seat in the unfolding drama and an up close and personal look at the local, state, and federal governmental response to COVID in his work with every state and territorial health official. He witnessed the impact of early efforts to slow the spread, the frustration that resulted from a lack of clarity in the federal response to COVID, and the confusing patchwork of state and territorial responses to the emerging virus. He saw the careers of colleagues and friends ended by public harassment and political retribution for the decisions they made to try to save lives by closing businesses and schools, and he experienced the lack of gubernatorial support for basic public health measures such as wearing face coverings and physical distancing that they recommended. He saw the stress, anger, and disappointment many state health officials experienced with shifting federal guidance, spotty public compliance, and the anxiety and worry health officials felt throughout the pandemic about the virus's spread, its potential lingering effects on health, the inequitable burden of disease in their communities, and waning support for efforts to protect the public from this novel pathogen.

And when a safe and effective vaccine did emerge, Fraser saw the sense of dismay and helplessness that spread as significant proportions of citizens rejected the vaccines they were freely offering to protect lives and restore livelihoods.

But he also saw great pride as state health officials put into action their plans to administer the lifesaving protection of safe and effective vaccines. He saw resilience in the face of tremendous adversity and a camaraderie emerge among our nation's health officials as strong as any between troops who had fought in a long, hard war. He gained an even deeper respect for their ability to lead diverse teams in a time of great stress, managing up, down, and across state and territorial government to protect the public's health. It was remarkable, unprecedented, and inspiring.

As a policy advisor to the Association of Immunization Managers, Brent Ewig saw up close the immense challenges that state and local public health professionals faced as they worked to transform and scale up a public health infrastructure previously focused on providing routine childhood vaccinations to serve an entire nation. As the intense work of planning turned to the early chaotic days of vaccine rollout, he saw the toll it was taking on these professionals. Six months into the vaccine distribution, he saw that a third of the 64 people who oversee the nation's vaccination programs had left as a result of either resignation, firing, or early retirement. This turnover was emblematic of the stress on the entire public health workforce and represented a startling loss of institutional knowledge when it was needed most. Despite this stress, seeing their work have such widespread lifesaving results has been a once-in-a-lifetime privilege.

At the onset of the pandemic, we both struggled to provide a collective voice to the resource needs of state health officials, their staff, and the communities they serve. This was especially needed when the Trump administration initially proposed a paltry $310 million, less than a dollar per person, to support the entire state and local effort to administer over 600 million doses of the new vaccine. While Congress would eventually direct over $6 billion to support the vaccination effort, the reality is that COVID vaccines arrived in states and communities before any significant resources arrived to assure it could efficiently get into arms.

Before COVID arrived, most Americans did not know who their state health official was. During COVID, and in the current post-acute phase of the pandemic, some state health officers have obtained celebrity status for their open, honest, and compassionate communication. Others have been vilified for their efforts to stop the virus that were perceived as restricting individual liberty, violating freedoms, or just another example of governmental overreach in the lives of everyday Americans. COVID response and the politics of disease prevention clouded nonpartisan attempts to end the pandemic. They spilled over into the national effort to vaccinate all eligible Americans and raised doubts about vaccine safety.

Never in our experience has the response to a public health threat caused such division. Vaccination, which could have been the single-easiest way to unite the country against COVID, became a political flash point.

This book covers the first 18 months of the largest vaccination campaign in modern American history: the effort to vaccinate America against SARS-CoV-2. By necessity, it should be viewed as a work in progress, since the story is not yet over. Yet the scope of the early campaign and the pressures surrounding it tell an important tale about politics and public health that informs the response to the current pandemic, as well as our potential response to emerging pathogens in the future.

Brian Tyler is the CEO of McKesson Corporation. His company, which was the centralized COVID vaccine distributor, was one of the most critical private-sector partners in the overall endeavor. In a documentary on McKesson's role in this historic process, he said:

I can remember driving down to the community center and getting my first dose of vaccine. Millions of people did that, but not a million people knew what it took to make that moment possible. Nobody saw the planning, nobody saw the building, nobody saw the training and the hiring, no one saw that team's commitment that made that miracle happen.[9]

As we honor partners like McKesson and so many others, we hope to help make the work he described visible.

And while the campaign could not have happened without the steadfast partnership of tens of thousands working in the private sector, including McKesson, FedEx, UPS, and vaccine manufacturers; workers in hospitals, clinics, CVS, Walgreens, and many other pharmacies; and pharmacists, doctors, nurses, and other clinicians, the core of this monumental effort was planned and executed by dedicated public servants in federal, state, and local public health and emergency management agencies and the US military. Together, these are the heroes who leapt into action to try to save lives.

This is a story that ultimately affects every human on the planet, and we acknowledge that at this point we do not know exactly how it ends. But this far into the effort, we have seen enough to share our impressions on what has worked and where we have fallen short. In the process, we want to raise up many of the unsung public health professionals who have worked past exhaustion. Especially at a time when trust in government is low, we feel it is important to celebrate the work of these public servants who have saved over two million lives.

We conclude this volume by identifying some of the lessons learned that matter the most and should be applied next time there is a pandemic event. The global conditions that allowed this previously unknown disease to emerge indicate that there almost surely will be a next time. These lessons, enumerated here, are about what matters:

1. Funding matters;
2. Trust matters;
3. Local, national, and global action matters;
4. Nonpartisanship matters; and
5. Leadership matters.

Tens of thousands of civil servants and public health professionals at the federal, state, and local levels have been working nearly nonstop for more than two years to turn vaccines into vaccinations in every corner of the nation. By sharing this story, we salute them all and want to make special mention of the 64 jurisdictional immunization program managers who serve as the lead official in their state responsible for eliminating vaccine-preventable diseases. We also salute the 59 chief state and territorial health officials who hold ultimate accountability for protecting the health of their fellow citizens, along with their incredible leadership teams. Together, these individuals have helped mobilize a public-private partnership to save lives unlike any other in American history.

There are certainly other volumes that detail the pandemic from many different vantage points, including insider tell-alls and leadership primers. This book is not meant to be either. Instead, we describe the COVID vaccination campaign from our experience working with and learning from state and territorial health officials and their leadership teams. Our experience is supplemented by interviews with over 20 individuals who have been on the front lines of this historic effort. This book attempts to give an inside look at what it meant to bring a rapidly developed COVID vaccine to the farthest reaches of our nation through the eyes of those who were tasked with doing it. While both celebrated and criticized, what state and territorial health officials, immunization program managers, and colleagues across the public health system were able to do in partnership with so many others had never before been accomplished at the speed and scale COVID required.

Theodore Roosevelt delivered a speech at the Sorbonne in Paris on April 23, 1910, that captures the spirit of this book. He stated:

> It is not the critic who counts; not the man who points out how the strong man stumbles, or where the doer of deeds could have done them better. The credit belongs to the man who is actually in the arena, whose face is marred by dust and sweat and blood; who strives valiantly; who errs, who comes short again and again, because there is no effort without error and shortcoming; but who does actually strive to do the deeds; who knows the great enthusiasms, the great devotions; who spends himself in a worthy cause; who at the best knows in the end the triumph of high achievement, and who at the worst, if he fails, at least fails while daring greatly, so that his place shall never be with those cold and timid souls who neither know victory nor defeat.[10]

We have been honored to work with the many people who made the COVID vaccination campaign their worthy cause. We too believe that tremendous credit is due to those in the COVID arena, the tireless public servants and partners who ran the race to vaccinate America together. While there have been failures, errors, and shortcomings along the way, all have dared greatly. And for that, we are extremely grateful.

Michael Fraser, PhD, MS
Brent Ewig, MHS
August 2022

REFERENCES

1. Taleb NN. Scaring us senseless. *New York Times*. July 24, 2005. Available at: https://www.nytimes.com/2005/07/24/opinion/scaring-us-senseless.html. Accessed September 13, 2022.
2. Santhanam L. Nurse who got first authorized US COVID vaccine: "we cannot continue to live like this." *PBS News Hour*. Public Broadcasting Service. December 14, 2021. Available at: https://www.pbs.org/newshour/health/sandra-lindsay-nurse-who-got-historic-covid-vaccine-reflects-on-omicron-and-whats-next. Accessed September 13, 2022.

3. Mitropoulos A. One year of COVID-19 vaccines: millions inoculated, but hundreds of thousands still lost. *ABC News.* December 14, 2021. Available at: https://abcnews.go.com/US/year-covid-19-vaccines-millions-inoculated-hundreds-thousands/story?id=81629912. Accessed September 13, 2022.

4. Schneider E, Shah A, Sah P, et al. Impact of US COVID-19 vaccination efforts: an update on averted deaths, hospitalizations, and health care costs through March 2022. The Commonwealth Fund. April 8, 2022. Available at: https://www.commonwealthfund.org/blog/2022/impact-us-covid-19-vaccination-efforts-march-update. Accessed September 13, 2022.

5. Centers for Disease Control and Prevention. United States COVID-19 cases and deaths by state over time. Available at: https://data.cdc.gov/Case-Surveillance/United-States-COVID-19-Cases-and-Deaths-by-State-o/9mfq-cb36. Accessed September 13, 2022.

6. Stephens T. *One Day at a Time: Newspapers and the Great Influenza of 1918.* Philadelphia, PA: Northern Liberties Press/Old City Publishing; 2021.

7. Painter WL. Tallying federal funding for COVID-19: in brief. Congressional Research Service. Updated October 15, 2021. Available at: https://crsreports.congress.gov/product/pdf/R/R46449. Accessed September 27, 2022.

8. Parlapiano A, Solomon DB, Ngo M, Cowley S. Where $5 trillion in pandemic stimulus money went. *New York Times.* March 11, 2022. Available at: https://www.nytimes.com/interactive/2022/03/11/us/how-covid-stimulus-money-was-spent.html. Accessed September 13, 2022.

9. McKesson. Standing ready: a documentary short. Available at: https://www.mckesson.com/About-McKesson/COVID-19-Documentary. Accessed September 13, 2022.

10. Theodore Roosevelt Center at Dickinson State University. The man in the arena. Available at: https://www.theodorerooseveltcenter.org/Learn-About-TR/TR-Encyclopedia/Culture-and-Society/Man-in-the-Arena.aspx. Accessed September 14, 2022.

Acknowledgments

Many colleagues and friends helped make this book possible. We thank Gregory Papillion for his research expertise and many contributions to the book's development as research associate. We also acknowledge the insights and expertise of the many professionals we interviewed as part of this project, including Claire Hannan, James Blumenstock, Molly Howell, Matthew Bobo, Michele Roberts, Stacy Hall, Bob Swanson, Dr. Rob Schechter, Dr. Walt Orenstein, Mitchel Rothholz, Dr. Kelly Moore, Dr. Tom Frieden, Adriane Casalotti, Paul Mango, Rebecca Coyle, Mary Beth Kurilo, and the individuals we spoke to who preferred to speak only on background. Their insights and experience were essential to shaping the story.

We also thank Carolyn Mullen, Senior Vice President for Public Relations and Government Affairs at ASTHO, for sharing key insights on public health advocacy and federal and state funding. We thank Sharon Miller, Senior Director for Governance at ASTHO, who helped piece together official statements and correspondence as part of our research. Several members of the ASTHO staff team were excellent sounding boards for ideas and issues covered in this book, including the staff of the Health Security Team. Many thanks to the team at APHA Press, including Daniel J. Doody, Maya Ribault, Ashell R. Alston, David Hartogs, cover designer Alan Giarcanella, and the team at KnowledgeWorks Gobal Ltd., including Cole Bowman and copyeditor Krystyna Budd. Thanks also to the many journalists, reporters, researchers, and authors whose works we cite in this volume. Their quick work and detailed reporting were indispensable in telling the COVID story as the virus emerged so quickly worldwide.

Brent would like to thank his family for their infinite patience and support throughout the preparation of this manuscript. Similarly, Michael appreciates the support of his family for their understanding and encouragement in the completion of this volume.

The opinions and statements expressed herein represent the personal viewpoints and perspectives of the authors and do not reflect the official policies or opinions of the Association of State and Territorial Health Officials and/or the Association of Immunization Managers or their individual members. Interviewee statements and other materials included in this volume should not be construed as endorsements by those individuals or organizations.

Readers' Note

Throughout this book, we use the term *COVID* to describe both the virus that causes COVID-19 disease (severe acute respiratory syndrome coronavirus 2, or SARS-CoV-2) and the disease itself (novel coronavirus disease or COVID, or COVID-19). While not exactly interchangeable, in most nonscientific literature on the novel coronavirus SARS-CoV-2 and COVID-19, using the term *COVID* for both the virus and its sequelae is standard practice. In the instances where the difference matters materially, we use SARS-CoV-2 to refer to the virus and COVID to refer to the disease caused by it.

In addition, there is debate over how to classify deaths attributable to COVID. Specifically, there is controversy over whether deaths that occurred *with* COVID (such as an individual who was admitted to a hospital for a stroke who was also infected with COVID) should be aggregated with deaths *from* COVID (an individual who died from illness related specifically to COVID).

There is also significant discussion on how to quantify deaths associated with individuals delaying care because they feared they could become infected with COVID while seeking care or treatment; or with an individual whose death is attributable to elective procedures (nonemergent care) being delayed for fear of becoming infected with COVID at health care systems strained by COVID; or with an individual whose death was caused by not being able to secure a hospital bed because of COVID cases overtaking hospital intensive care units; or with deaths caused by individuals not seeking care because they lost health insurance when employment ended as a result of COVID restrictions or even because the costs of COVID-related treatment were unaffordable. Whenever it is possible to discern the exact nature of the way deaths are reported, the specific term (*from* or *with*) is stated. However, where it is unclear if deaths include *from*, *with*, or otherwise because of COVID-related barriers, we use the phrase *deaths from COVID* broadly.

A Perfect Storm

We have it totally under control. It's one person coming in from China, and we have it under control. It's going to be just fine.[1]

–President Trump, January 22, 2020

Disruption to everyday life might be severe.[2]

–Dr. Nancy Messonnier, Centers for Disease Control
and Prevention, February 25, 2020

We know these measures will significantly disrupt people's day-to-day lives, but they are absolutely necessary. This is going to be a defining moment for our city and we all have a responsibility to do our part to protect our neighbors and slow the spread of this virus by staying at home unless it is absolutely essential to go outside.[3]

–London Breed, Mayor of San Francisco, first US city to announce
shelter-in-place order, March 16, 2020

I hope this marks the beginning of the end of a very painful time in our history.[4]

–Nurse Sandra Lindsay upon receiving the first US COVID vaccination
outside of clinical trials on December 14, 2020

America's health was at risk well before the novel coronavirus we now call COVID spread exponentially into a global pandemic in early 2020. Our collective political health was at risk: America was bitterly divided along partisan lines and about to embark on a contentious presidential election. Our collective physical and mental health were also at risk: American life expectancy at birth began to decline in 2017, after 50 years of steady increases, and continued to decrease every year thereafter with persistent and significant gaps between white and non-white Americans across the board.[5]

The health of the nation's governmental public health agencies was also at risk: the local and state governmental public health system rooted in federalism and a confusing set of local, state, and federal laws, regulations, and funding sources was already strained before COVID and became even more so as the pandemic unfolded. This was the system that would be called on to conduct the largest and most complex public health campaign in American history.

At the start of 2020, public health agencies were overtaxed by increasing rates of addiction, suicide, and overdose deaths, in addition to growing rates of chronic disease, sexually transmitted infections, regional outbreaks of preventable communicable diseases such as pertussis and measles, increasing vector-borne diseases, and the health effects of climate-related extreme weather events and natural disasters. Responding to a global pandemic is no easy feat, but COVID's emergence at a particularly inauspicious time in America's history made the public health response even more difficult. And yet, despite the fragile state of our nation's public health departments and the myriad barriers that public health leaders needed to overcome to implement the largest and most successful vaccine distribution campaign in American history, they did it. Before we turn to the specifics of the campaign, it is important to introduce the broader context in which the massive vaccine effort was planned and executed.

WARP SPEED AHEAD

New Year's Day 2020 ushered in a global pandemic and a chaotic, uncoordinated first few months of mixed messages about the novel coronavirus. Top political leaders and federal officials first downplayed the risk of any severe health impacts of COVID, then quickly did an about-face and stressed COVID's severity and the need for shutdowns to slow the spread as more was learned about the virus's impact. The US federal government first focused on travel bans and repatriation of overseas citizens as the pandemic unfolded, but by mid-March 2020, when community transmission of COVID was established in the United States, officials urged citizens to stay at home; closed businesses at which people gathered such as movie theaters, restaurants, and gyms; prohibited large gatherings; and closed schools and day care centers to prevent community spread. As Dr. Nancy Messonnier, former director of the National Center for Immunization and Respiratory Diseases, a division of the Centers for Disease Control and Prevention (CDC), and now dean of the University of North Carolina Gillings School of Public Health, predicted in her February 25, 2020, remarks on a CDC COVID media telebriefing, disruptions to everyday life were indeed severe.[2]

After a spring of shutdowns, the US Food and Drug Administration (FDA) approval of rapid antigen tests, and emerging scientific consensus on the effectiveness of face coverings in preventing aerosolized transmission of COVID, the summer of 2020 was characterized by messages from those eager to quickly reopen and "liberate" states from pandemic lockdowns while many public health officials stressed continued caution, masking, and social distancing.

Operation Warp Speed was launched on May 15, 2020, amid this chaos, with an initial $10 billion taxpayer investment in vaccines and therapeutics to combat COVID. The warp speed moniker was chosen as a nod to the need for the speedy creation of a COVID vaccine but immediately raised questions about the safety of its rapid development and review. These questions churned in the press and social media amid the turmoil of America's early COVID response and an amped-up election season, led by a president intensely interested in sustaining a robust economy and developing a vaccine before a looming November election. The Trump administration promised to expedite vaccine development and approval, which is traditionally a painstakingly detailed, multistage, and multiple-year effort. This reflected the urgency of developing safe and effective vaccines, but the focus on speed seeded mistrust of the industries manufacturing the vaccines and the regulatory agencies charged with protecting the public in the process.

STORM CLOUDS GATHER: FEDERALISM AND PUBLIC HEALTH IN AMERICA

Meteorologists use the expression *perfect storm* to describe a weather event that results from a combination of unusual meteorological patterns that align to create a rare and powerful tempest. COVID's rapid emergence from a novel pathogen first reported to the World Health Organization on December 31, 2019,[6] to a global pandemic on March 11, 2020,[7] struck an already unhealthy America and grew exponentially. COVID's landfall in the United States was a perfect storm in which a previously unknown virus met an underresourced and understaffed public health system in a nation riddled by growing vaccine skepticism and distrust of government.

The storm laid bare long-standing racial and ethnic inequities and glaring holes in our social safety net. It became an even more dangerous storm when politicized by those who pitted the reopening of the economy against protecting the public's health to score points in a turbulent election season. As Dr. Deborah Birx, former White House Coronavirus Task Force coordinator, rightly stated on *Face the Nation* soon after her retirement from federal service in January 2021, "The worst possible time you can have a pandemic is in a presidential election year."[8]

Planning an unprecedented national immunization program occurred against a backdrop of conspiracy theories about COVID's origin and concerns about the speed of vaccine development; racial upheaval and turmoil as a result of the murder of George Floyd in the summer of 2020; an attempt by outgoing president Donald Trump, radicalized Republicans, and white supremacists to overthrow the US Congress's certification of President-Elect Joe Biden's election victory at the Capitol on January 6, 2021; and an anti-science narrative that COVID was a hoax. Despite these headwinds, the US public health system and its partners delivered over 500 million doses of COVID vaccine to the American people in less than a year.[9] This unprecedented achievement provided protection against severe illness, hospitalization, and death to 67% of fully vaccinated Americans age six months or older, or 222.3 million Americans as of July 1, 2022.[9]

On a good day, public health in America operates in the background. To most Americans, the governmental public health system is invisible, although all of us benefit from its many functions. Safe drinking water, clean air, newborn screening for inheritable diseases, communicable disease reporting and follow-up, tobacco purchase and use restrictions to minors, maternal and child health programs, food outbreak investigations and food safety inspections, health facilities regulations, birth and death registrations, and many other functions are common to most public health agencies and operated by all state and local public health authorities.

Routine public health activities often go unnoticed: when nothing happens that could impact the public's health, a health officer can rest easy. Public health advocates point out that it is only when a crisis occurs that the public pays heed to what governmental public health agencies do, most often during large outbreaks and environmental disasters. COVID was such a crisis, thrusting the work of local, state, and federal governmental public health agencies into the daily news, which became fodder for commendation as well as critique and contention.

To fully understand the US response to COVID and the challenges in rolling out a vaccination campaign of the scale and speed required, it is vital to understand the way governmental public health agencies operate nationwide. Unlike countries with health systems and governmental public health agencies that are centralized in a national system, the public health system in the United States is decentralized. America's public health system comprises over 3,000 health agencies at the local, state, tribal, and territorial levels, all with differing structures, capabilities, and capacities. Some states have local public health agencies that operate under the authority of the state health departments; others have decentralized and autonomous county and city public health agencies. Vast areas of some states have no local public health authorities. The creation of public health departments is largely the result of the way state and local governments were established across an expanding geographic territory early in our history. Unlike most US health care delivery, which is privately run by large nonprofit and for-profit health systems and hospital corporations, the protection of the public's health is a governmental responsibility, not a market function. The provision of population-wide, community-based public health services has traditionally been the purview of states and territories, not the federal government, and states have approached this work differently on the basis of their populations, politics, and state resources. Moreover, their relationships with local officials vary widely.

The US Constitution's specific charge for states to protect the health of their residents is rooted in its delegation of police powers to the states. Public health legal scholar Lawrence Gostin explains as follows:

> The Constitution allocates public health powers among the federal government and the states. Federal public health powers include the authority to tax, spend, and regulate interstate commerce. These powers enable the federal government to raise revenues, allocate resources, economically penalize risk behavior, and broadly regulate in the public's interest. . . . States have an inherent authority to protect, preserve, and promote the health, safety, morals, and general welfare of the people, termed *police powers*. Police powers enable states to preserve the public health in areas ranging from injury and disease prevention to sanitation, waste disposal, and environmental protection.[10(p2979)]

This policy supports the authority of local and state health officers to protect the public's health by issuing containment and mitigation orders, including business closures, mandating vaccinations for school entry, limiting crowd size, and requiring face coverings indoors to prevent infections and disease transmission. In typical operations, a health officer may quarantine a resident with tuberculosis or close a food establishment for sanitary violations.

To prevent COVID transmission and infection, public health authority had to be exercised broadly and health officers issued stay-at-home and masking orders for entire communities. Given the low visibility of public health agencies' work before COVID compared to other government services such as police and fire departments, the exercise of significant police powers of state and local public health officers came as a surprise to many. Emerging alongside their governors in press conferences and media appearances, state and territorial health officials were thrust into the limelight. The public quickly became aware of what their local and state public health agencies do, and as with many things in America in 2020, seemingly half the population approved, but half the population did not.

The delegation of health protection to individual states, along with the diversity of funding streams that support governmental public health activities, created significant tensions between local, state, and federal response efforts to COVID. Many pundits and members of the public decried inconsistent and uncoordinated state and county public health actions and called for a more centralized, uniform, and consistent governmental response to COVID. But these calls ignored the long-standing law and practice of American federalism that has guided state-federal interactions and authorities since the founding of our nation.

Why, some asked, would restaurants be open in one state but not in a neighboring state? Why would masks be required in some schools but not in all districts? Why would proof of vaccination be required in some cities but not in others? How can some governors reopen their economies, while others continue to lock them down? These questions also underscored how most Americans lack awareness of the nature of our nation's federal-state system and the role of government in promoting and protecting the public's health. Rather than creating an environment where all Americans felt we were in the COVID struggle together, inconsistencies created confusion and reduced trust in both government and science. This confusion and concerns about public health's authority would later significantly impact the nascent COVID vaccine distribution program.

The public health powers of the federal government extend primarily to the protection of national borders and ports of entry and federal property and to the regulation of interstate commerce (i.e., masking in federal buildings, in airports, and on interstate conveyances). Almost three years into a pandemic, the ability of the president of the United States to issue broad protective orders in a national public health emergency, such as ordering a federal mask mandate applicable to all states or requiring nonfederal employers to vaccinate their workforces, has been largely blocked by federal courts.

Federalism does not mean states are on their own in a national emergency or that the federal government sits idly by as states respond to public health disasters. For federalism to work as intended, there must be an active partnership and coordinated action between the federal government and other units of government that allows for local variation in policy setting and decision-making.

The original authors of the US Constitution were wary of strong central control and promoted checks and balances to assure that governmental decision-making was rooted in local authority (landowning white men), not central authority (a king). The US Constitution never mentions the word *health*, but it does authorize Congress to "make all Laws which shall be necessary and proper" to carry out its mandate "to . . . provide for . . . general Welfare."[11] The result is the diverse set of authorities and responsibilities that characterize the nation's local, state, territorial, tribal, and federal public health system. Importantly, this diversity of approaches and state and local control is baked into our constitutional system and does not change in a pandemic, a fact that many talk show pundits, members of the public, and even some politicians failed to grasp when calling for more, or less, federal government action in the COVID response.

Preparedness and response planning at the federal level generally refers to how federal departments and agencies coordinate with and support state, territorial, local, and tribal partners in a variety of ways during a public health emergency or event of national significance. Planning assumptions before COVID were generally based on an emerging disease threat that starts overseas and is gradually introduced to the United States through infected international travelers who transmit a virus, such as influenza or Ebola, domestically and present at a local hospital or health care provider. Federal plans include working with local and state leaders to assess how federal assets will be used to quarantine travelers and support the continuing operations of the federal government in an emergency. The plans also outline ways the federal government will assist governors and mayors when their jurisdictions are overwhelmed by a disaster or there is a need to quickly procure at scale the resources all states may need in a response, such as therapeutics, ventilators, personal protective equipment, or, as is the focus of this book, vaccines.

Agencies such as the US Department of Health and Human Services (HHS) and its component agencies, including the CDC, typically conduct pandemic and public health emergency planning scenarios and exercise plans with many response partners to review planning assumptions. They also meet with state, territorial, and local partners to conduct after-action review of actual public health events and disasters. The resulting after-action reports share several consistent themes on these actual events and fictional exercises, including Crimson Contagion, an August 2019 scenario-based exercise with federal, state, and local partners conducted just four months before COVID was first reported.[12] These themes include variations on the following findings: there will be insufficient federal funding for necessary response activities; confusion will reign over who is in charge of the response at the federal, state, and local levels; getting real-time data from public health and health care agencies will be difficult, as will aggregating it nationally; and the capacity of state and local health agencies will quickly be overwhelmed as infections increase.

Reports have also found that existing mechanisms to gather situational awareness or ground truth to inform state and national action are insufficient; that mechanisms to coordinate action among states and between states and the federal government are often developed ad hoc, resulting in inadequate collaboration to meet the demands of the crisis; that communities of color and non-English-speaking communities are frequently left out of planning and response efforts; that plans for people with disabilities are generally deficient because they fail to address the complexity of that population; and that tribal jurisdictions and remote US territories in the Atlantic and Pacific are often omitted entirely in national planning efforts. Each of these themes would play out in the planning and execution of the COVID vaccine program as well.

Previous playbooks and exercises designed to guide state and federal responses in public health emergencies generally assume that the HHS secretary, in conjunction with the HHS assistant secretary for preparedness and response and the CDC director, would provide significant national leadership in consultation with the White House and other government agencies and would work in partnership with state and local health leaders. Indeed, following that playbook, CDC director Dr. Robert Redfield made HHS secretary Alex Azar aware of the novel coronavirus emergency in China in late December 2019 and early January 2020.[13] But as the pandemic progressed and the COVID response became increasingly partisan, leadership moved from the CDC, to HHS, to the White House and its COVID Task Force, briefly led by Secretary Azar, who was replaced by Vice President Pence, who then announced the appointment of Dr. Deborah Birx as task force coordinator in late February 2020.[14]

Because an effective national response to a pandemic depends on the ability of state and territorial health agencies to implement appropriate disease control and prevention measures in active collaboration with the federal government, one would imagine the need for current or former state or territorial health officials to help advise federal leaders on a routine, predecisional and deliberative basis. Whereas state and territorial health officials were in constant contact with CDC colleagues and some HHS staff about the tactical work of COVID response, there was limited collaboration on COVID policy between the White House Coronavirus Task Force and state health officers early in the pandemic response. State health officers would often learn about policy changes and recommendations decided by the White House from the media or from their governors, who would be briefed just hours before significant developments or changes were announced.

Frustrated by the lack of engagement in predecisional, deliberative policy discussions, professional organizations representing state and local public health leaders, including the Association of State and Territorial Health Officials and the National Association of County and City Health Officials, repeatedly called for the establishment of better communication at the leadership level between the Trump administration and their members. Unfortunately, however, such improvements never took place.

The dynamic of federal policy setting by press release gave state and local public health officials limited to no opportunity to discuss implementation challenges or state and local perspectives before their announcement, including substantive discussions about vaccine development and planning for vaccine rollout. The failure of the White House Coronavirus Task Force and many HHS leaders to specifically engage state and territorial public health officials early in the pandemic created missed opportunities for the White House and HHS leaders to work directly with those who were attempting to align state efforts and governors' priorities with federal policy whenever possible.

Andy Slavitt, the acting administrator of the Centers for Medicare and Medicaid Services in the Obama administration and volunteer adviser to the Trump administration's early COVID response, highlights what might be one reason for the lack of intentional engagement of state and local public health leaders in deliberations on COVID policy. In his book *Preventable: The Inside Story of How Leadership Failures, Politics, and Selfishness Doomed the US Coronavirus Response*, Slavitt recounts the attitude of some White House officials and advisers to the president who, rather than viewing states as partners in the shared work of COVID response, might have been holding states at bay so that they could serve as scapegoats for any COVID response failures.[15] Slavitt describes Trump's penchant to avoid accountability at any cost, which is exemplified in his infamous "I don't take responsibility at all,"[16] a response to questions about the Trump administration's missteps in producing an accurate test for COVID in March 2020. This was followed by "it is what it is,"[17] made in response to the US milestone of 1,000 COVID-related deaths a day in July 2020, and then the contradictory "I take full responsibility. It's not my fault that it came here. It's China's fault,"[18] a comment made at the October 22, 2020, presidential debate with Joe Biden in Nashville, Tennessee.

Federalism requires a robust partnership between federal and state governments that was sorely tested and found lacking throughout the COVID response. In many ways, Slavitt was right. Rather than acknowledging federalism and the need for strong federal-state-local partnership, states were often used to deflect blame for the administration's missteps and lack of clarity on response goals. Trump summed it up in a teleconference call with governors on April 16, 2020, in which he told them bluntly, "You are going to call your own shots,"[19] referring to state decision-making on reopening criteria and social distancing and gathering restrictions. This statement was made despite the administration's release six days later of its *Guidelines for Opening Up America Again* document, which set recommended gating criteria for states to use to "help state and local officials when reopening their economies, getting people back to work, and continuing to protect American lives."[20]

At a White House briefing a few days before the official release of the *Guidelines* document, Trump stated, "We will hold the governors accountable. But again, we're going to be working with them to make sure it works very well."[21] What, exactly, the White House was holding governors accountable for was not made explicit. States' adoption of the White House plan was mixed, with many governors opting to create their own metrics and benchmarks for lifting restrictions in consultation with their health officers, not federal officials. There ensued super-spreader events—large gatherings where multiple persons were infected with COVID—and these led to a predicted increase of COVID cases across the southeastern states and COVID's second wave later in the summer of 2020.[22]

The opportunity to create shared national messages to inform Americans on the collective risks posed by a virus that could be spread asymptomatically and to help foster a shared sense of social cohesion, community, and responsibility was missed. Instead, the newfound freedom to infect your neighbors with COVID by not wearing masks, nor social distancing, was celebrated as a victory for personal liberty by many. Harassment of health officials increased;[23] and as governors and state legislators reacted to constituents' anger toward public health mandates and lockdowns, legislative attempts to undermine public health authority began in earnest.[24,25] On-the-fly efforts to balance personal freedoms and economic progress with public health protections created wide variability in COVID mitigation tactics among states. To some, this was federalism at its best, but to many others it was federalism at its worst.

The one thing it seemed most local, state, and federal leaders could agree on was the urgent need to administer the newly developed COVID vaccines to the American public as quickly as possible. The successful development of vaccines to protect against severe disease from COVID infection and to potentially limit transmission of the virus overall was the most significant success in the first year of the COVID response. This scientific achievement and the eventual development of rapid antigen testing for COVID, along with new antiviral and monoclonal antibody therapeutics to reduce disease severity or prevent infection, were game changers in the nation's campaign against COVID. The distribution and administration of these vaccines—that is, turning a vaccine into a vaccination—would test federalism again by requiring tremendous state and federal collaboration, along with the collaboration of the private sector, health care and hospitals leaders, and thousands of community groups and local leaders.

The Biden administration took over at a key moment in the nation's COVID response, just 37 days after the first COVID vaccination was administered in the United States. Key to the new administration's approach was active consultation among federal, state, and local health officials, particularly around the emerging vaccine campaign. The new administration's White House COVID Task Force quickly set up weekly, if not more frequent, teleconferences between state and local health officials and public health professional organizations. These included CDC and other HHS officials as well as the White House COVID Task Force leadership, whose aim was to share information and inform policies.

In a significant and much-needed policy move, the Biden administration and Congress proposed crucial new investments for the nation's local, state, and federal public health infrastructure to sustain needed improvements that had been identified in the first year of COVID response. These included proposed investments in workforce expansion, data systems improvement, and support for efforts to address health equity across the country to ensure that all Americans had access to vaccines for COVID and other public health and health care services in the future.[26,27] These investments would help state and local health officials carry out the immediate challenge of COVID response and help build much-needed public health capacity for future public health activities.

BEFORE THE STORM: PUBLIC HEALTH CAPACITY IN THE UNITED STATES PRE-COVID

COVID demonstrated the wide variation in workforce capacity, information technology capacity, and other limitations of a public health system that lost staff and resources during the Great Recession in 2009 and never recovered. State and local public health agencies entered 2020 with fewer workers than they had in 2009 and with legacy information technology and data systems that had been in place for decades.[28] Local public health departments lost 55,000 jobs between 2008 and 2017 as their budgets fell by a quarter.[29,30] During that same period, state health agencies lost almost 20,000 jobs, and between 2010 and 2018 funding dropped by 22%.[31,32] According to a 2022 report by the Public Health National Center for Innovations, over 80,000 new public health workers are needed to be able to adequately staff the core functions of governmental public health agencies at the local, state, and territorial levels nationwide in addition to the almost 90,000 state and territorial health agency staff that are employed today.[33]

Fighting a global pandemic at the national level requires finding the balance between a strong centralized response that allows for state and local variability. Beefing up state public health capacity had to be accomplished expeditiously to respond to the exponentially increasing threat of COVID. This required quick action to hire new workers, procure needed services and supplies, and expand administrative operations in real time. Federal assets, also strained, had to be quickly and equitably deployed to state and local public health agencies to support the response. Processes to achieve this balance between state and federal capabilities had been built into the HHS pandemic plans of both the Bush and the Obama administrations, but the Trump administration refused to follow anyone else's playbook. As we describe later, the White House sidelined the HHS and CDC officials with the most experience in fighting infectious disease, vacillated in the administration's approach to federalism, and often questioned state needs for additional resources. All these factors cast a shadow over COVID vaccine distribution and administration plans.

There are, however, several critical public health functions that all states receive CDC funding to support, and one of these areas is immunization. For decades, every state and territorial health agency has received grants from the CDC that provide core funding for the nation's immunization services through a program known as the Section 317 Immunization Program (Section 317 Program), awkwardly named for the section of the Public Health Service Act that authorizes it. The program is administered by the Immunization Services Division of the CDC's National Center for Immunization and Respiratory Disease, the same entity that manages the Vaccines for Children (VFC) program,[34] a federally funded entitlement program created in 1993 that complements the Section 317 Program by providing vaccines at no cost to children who might not otherwise be vaccinated because of inability to pay. It was developed after earlier efforts to develop a federal universal vaccine purchase program were unsuccessful. Under VFC, the CDC buys vaccine at a discounted rate for centralized distribution to registered VFC providers. Whereas VFC funding is automatically determined by need, public health advocates note that Section 317 Program funding has been stagnant for at least the past decade. Nevertheless, this program did provide the foundational capabilities and critical infrastructure for state and local COVID vaccine distribution. Sustainable and adequate funding for both immunization and broader public health infrastructure had, however, been an ongoing challenge well before the COVID pandemic.

In a January 2022 presentation to the HHS Health Information Technology Advisory Committee, former CDC director Thomas (Tom) Frieden described expecting the US public health system to have effectively responded to COVID as akin to expecting someone with their feet encased in concrete to swim.[35] Given the diverse and decentralized system that delivers public health services across the country, that analogy may be quite accurate. Indeed, at the outset of planning the greatest and most complex vaccine campaign in American history, the governmental public health system was battling a perfect storm of underfunding, understaffing, and a confusing system of local, state, and federal authorities. It is a testament to the dedication, skill, and tenacity of our country's public health professionals that despite this storm they succeeded in vaccinating the nation.

In a February 2022 article in *STAT News*, health care journalist Helen Branswell calls the development, production, and administration of COVID vaccines a "freaking miracle."[36] Indeed, the fact that our nation's public health system ably scaled up and transformed to meet the challenges of vaccinating America during an unprecedented global pandemic seems like a "freaking miracle" as well. The massive public-private effort to both develop vaccines and then get them into arms is unprecedented. While nothing could prepare the public health system for the magnitude of the undertaking and the thousands of details administering new vaccines would require, lessons from previous pandemics informed planning efforts and provided key insights to those willing to learn from them.

REFERENCES

1. Summers J. Timeline: how Trump has downplayed the coronavirus pandemic. National Public Radio. October 2, 2020. Available at: https://www.npr.org/sections/latest-updates-trump-covid-19-results/2020/10/02/919432383/how-trump-has-downplayed-the-coronavirus-pandemic. Accessed September 13, 2022.

2. Centers for Disease Control and Prevention. Transcript for the CDC telebriefing update on COVID-19. [Press briefing transcript]. February 26, 2020. Available at: https://www.cdc.gov/media/releases/2020/t0225-cdc-telebriefing-covid-19.html. Accessed September 13, 2022.

3. Office of the Mayor. San Francisco issues new public health order requiring residents stay at home except for essential needs. [News release]. March 16, 2020. Available at: https://sfmayor.org/article/san-francisco-issues-new-public-health-order-requiring-residents-stay-home-except-essential. Accessed September 13, 2022.

4. Covid-19: first vaccine given in US as roll-out begins. *BBC News*. December 14, 2020. Available at: https://www.bbc.com/news/world-us-canada-55305720. Accessed September 13, 2022.

5. Arias E, Tejada-Vera B, Ahmad F, Kochanek KD. Provisional life expectancy estimates for 2020. Vital Statistics Rapid Release; no 15. Hyattsville, MD: National Center for Health Statistics; July 2021. doi:10.15620/cdc:107201.

6. World Health Organization. Pneumonia of unknown cause—China. January 5, 2020. Available at: https://www.who.int/emergencies/disease-outbreak-news/item/2020-DON229. Accessed September 13, 2022.

7. Cucinotta D, Vanelli M. WHO declares COVID-19 a pandemic. *Acta Biomed*. 2020 2020;91(1):157–160. doi:10.23750/abm.v91i1.9397.

8. CBS News. Transcript: Dr. Deborah Birx on "Face the Nation," January 24, 2021. Available at: https://www.cbsnews.com/news/transcript-deborah-birx-on-face-the-nation-january-24-2021. Accessed September 13, 2022.

9. Centers for Disease Control and Prevention. CDC COVID data tracker. Available at: https://covid.cdc.gov/covid-data-tracker/#datatracker-home. Accessed September 13, 2022.

10. Gostin L. Public health law in a new century, II: public health powers and limits. *JAMA*. 2000;283(22):2979–2984.

11. Legal Information Institute. Necessary and proper clause. Available at: https://www.law.cornell.edu/wex/necessary_and_proper_clause. Accessed September 13, 2022.

12. US Department of Health and Human Services. Office of the Assistant Secretary for Preparedness and Response. Crimson contagion 2019 functional exercise after-action report. January 2020. Available at: https://www.governmentattic.org/38docs/HHSaarCrimsonContAAR_2020.pdf. Accessed September 13, 2022.

13. Woodward B. *Rage*. New York, NY: Simon & Schuster; 2021.

14. Kaiser Family Foundation. VP Pence announces appointment of Ambassador Deborah Birx as White House coronavirus response coordinator. February 28, 2020. Available at:

https://www.kff.org/news-summary/vp-pence-announces-appointment-of-ambassador-deborah-birx-as-white-house-coronavirus-response-coordinator. Accessed September 13, 2022.

15. Slavitt A. *Preventable: The Inside Story of How Leadership Failures, Politics, and Selfishness Doomed the US Coronavirus Response*. New York: St. Martin's Press; 2021.

16. Oprusko C. "I don't take responsibility at all": Trump deflects blame for coronavirus testing fumble. *Politico*. March 13, 2020. Available at: https://www.politico.com/news/2020/03/13/trump-coronavirus-testing-128971. Accessed September 13, 2022.

17. Shabad R. 'It is what it is": Trump in interview on COVID-19 death toll in US. *NBC News*. August 4, 2020. Available at: https://www.nbcnews.com/politics/donald-trump/it-what-it-trump-interview-covid-19-death-toll-u-n1235734. Accessed September 13, 2022.

18. Lopez G. Trump on Covid-19: "I take full responsibility. it's not my fault." *Vox*. October 22, 2020. Available at: https://www.vox.com/future-perfect/2020/10/22/21529666/debate-trump-biden-coronavirus-responsibility-fault. Accessed September 14, 2022.

19. O'Keefe E, Watson K. "You're gonna call your own shots," Trump tells governors about guidelines to reopen states. *CBS News*. Updated April 16, 2020. Available at: https://www.cbsnews.com/news/trump-guidelines-on-opening-up-america-leave-much-up-to-governors. Accessed September 13, 2022.

20. National Archives and Records Administration. Guidelines: opening up America again. Available at: https://trumpwhitehouse.archives.gov/openingamerica. Accessed September 14, 2022.

21. Remarks by President Trump in press briefing, April 14, 2020. The White House. April 14, 2020. Available at: https://it.usembassy.gov/remarks-by-president-trump-in-press-briefing-april-14-2020. Accessed September 13, 2022.

22. Coccia M. The impact of first and second wave of the COVID-19 pandemic in society: comparative analysis to support control measures to cope with negative effects of future infectious diseases. *Environ Res*. 2021;197:111099. doi:10.1016/j.envres.2021.111099.

23. Fraser MR. Harassment of health officials: a significant threat to the public's health. *Amer J Public Health*. 2022;112(5):728–730. doi:10.2105/ajph.2022.306797.

24. Association of State and Territorial Health Officials. Maintaining public health's legal authority to prevent disease spread. Available at: https://www.astho.org/globalassets/pdf/legislative-prospectus_public-health-authority.pdf. Accessed September 13, 2022.

25. National Association of County and City Health Officials. Proposed limits on public health authority: dangerous for public health. May 2021. Available at: https://www.naccho.org/uploads/downloadable-resources/Proposed-Limits-on-Public-Health-Authority-Dangerous-for-Public-Health-FINAL-5.24.21pm.pdf. Accessed September 13, 2022.

26. The White House. Biden–Harris administration to invest $7 billion from American rescue plan to hire and train public health workers in response to COVID-19. [Fact sheet]. May 13, 2021. Available at: https://www.whitehouse.gov/briefing-room/statements-releases/2021/05/13/fact-sheet. Accessed September 14, 2022.

27. Kates J, Wexler A. Public health infrastructure and pandemic preparedness provisions in the Build Back Better Act. Kaiser Family Foundation. November 10, 2021. Available at: https://www.kff.org/coronavirus-covid-19/issue-brief/public-health-infrastructure-and-pandemic-preparedness-provisions-in-the-build-back-better-act. Accessed September 14, 2022.

28. Association of State and Territorial Health Officials. ASTHO profile of state and territorial public health, volume 4. Available at: https://www.astho.org/globalassets/pdf/profile/profile-stph-vol-4.pdf. Accessed September 13, 2022.

29. National Association of County and City Health Officials. NACCHO's 2019 profile study: changes in local health department workforce and finance capacity since 2008. [Research brief]. May 2020. Available at: https://www.naccho.org/blog/articles/naccho-new-analysis-changes-in-local-health-department-workforce-and-finance-capacity-since-2008. Accessed September 24, 2022.

30. Trust for America's Health. The impact of chronic underfunding on America's public health system: trends, risks, and recommendations, 2019. April 2019. Available at: https://www.tfah.org/wp-content/uploads/2020/03/TFAH_2019_PublicHealthFunding_07.pdf. Accessed September 24, 2022.

31. Weber L, Ungar L, Smith MR. Hollowed-out public health system faces more cuts amid virus. *Kaiser Health News*. Updated August 24, 2020. Available at: https://khn.org/news/us-public-health-system-underfunded-under-threat-faces-more-cuts-amid-covid-pandemic. Accessed September 13, 2022.

32. Trust for America's Health and the Coalition for Health Funding. Congressional briefing and national webinar: beyond emergency funding: sustaining public health funding in the post-COVID landscape. June 22, 2022. Available at: https://www.tfah.org/wp-content/uploads/2022/06/TFAH_CHF_Public_Health_Funding_Congressional_Briefing.pdf. Accessed September 13, 2022.

33. Public Health National Center for Innovations. Staffing up: governmental public health workforce calculator. Available at: https://phnci.org/national-frameworks/staffing-up. Accessed September 13, 2022.

34. Jarris P, Dolen V. Section 317 Immunization Program: protecting a national asset. *Public Health Rep*. 2013;128(2):96–98. doi:10.1177/003335491312800204.

35. Frieden T. Public health system performance during COVID-19. The Office of the National Coordinator for Health Information Technology. May 13, 2021. Available at: https://www.healthit.gov/sites/default/files/facas/2021-05-13_Tom_Frieden_508.pdf. Accessed September 24, 2022.

36. Branswell H. Why COVID-19 vaccines are a freaking miracle. *STAT*. February 14, 2022. Available at: https://www.statnews.com/2022/02/14/why-covid-19-vaccines-are-a-freaking-miracle. Accessed August 12, 2022.

2

What Is Past Is Prologue

The success of the pandemic influenza vaccination program will be determined in large part by the strength of state and local vaccination programs during the Interpandemic Period.[1]

–HHS Influenza Pandemic Plan,
November 2005

There's one thing that I can tell you about this: It [COVID] is much more aggressive in its transmission than anything that we have seen in recent history . . . It is probably more akin to the 1918 pandemic.[2]

–Senator Richard Burr, Chairman, Senate Intelligence Committee,
February 27, 2020

Well before COVID, earlier pandemics tested America's resolve and public health agencies' response capacity. These pandemics, while thankfully rare, required governmental public health agencies to respond in multiple ways, including deploying vaccines as medical countermeasures when available. The most recent pandemic, the 2009 H1N1 influenza outbreak, required the mobilization of a national vaccine program by federal, state, and local governmental health agencies. While COVID vaccine planning was based on many of the planning assumptions and response lessons learned in these past responses, much of the Trump administration's Operation Warp Speed campaign also deviated from past approaches. This chapter provides a brief review of the role of vaccines in past pandemic responses and the planning in place prior to the emergence of COVID.

THE ROLE OF VACCINES IN EARLIER PANDEMICS

The classic definition of a pandemic is "an epidemic occurring worldwide, or over a very wide area, crossing international boundaries and usually affecting a large number of people."[3] If a new microbe can infect humans and achieve human-to-human transmission, a pandemic may arise because humans are unlikely to have immunity to the new virus. Where available, vaccines can quickly provide that immunity and help end pandemics.

In the century before COVID, four pandemics were caused by the emergence of a novel influenza strain for which humans possessed little or no immunity: the H1N1 Spanish flu (1918), the H2N2 Asian flu (1957), the H3N2 Hong Kong flu (1968), and the H1N1 swine flu (2009). The most devastating pandemic in modern history was the

1918–1919 influenza outbreak, with an estimated 675,000 deaths in the United States and 50 million worldwide.[4] The only global pandemic that may have claimed more lives is the Bubonic Plague that swept Europe, Asia, and North Africa in the 1300s.[5]

The 1918–1919 flu pandemic occurred during World War I, which likely facilitated its spread and in which the historically linked dangers of warfare and disease took a devastating toll. In her article "The US Military and the Influenza Pandemic of 1918–1919," Dr. Carol Byerly reports that influenza and pneumonia killed more US troops in World War I than enemy weapons.[6] Byerly further notes:

> World War I and influenza collaborated: the war fostered disease by creating conditions in the trenches of France that some epidemiologists believe enabled the influenza virus to evolve into a killer of global proportions. In turn, disease shaped the war effort by rendering much of the Army and Navy *non-effective* and diverting resources, personnel, and scarce human attention and energy from the military campaign [emphasis added].[6]

Over 56,000 American soldiers are estimated to have died from the disease in 1918 as compared to 53,402 killed in combat.[7]

In his epic volume *The Great Influenza*, author John Barry recounts the inability of scientists to identify the pathogen causing the 1918 pandemic, which effectively prevented the development of a viable vaccine to prevent it.[8] While there were some heroic but scattershot attempts to develop a vaccine, they were not widely available and had decidedly mixed results.[9] It would be another 15 years before the virus that causes influenza was identified, but the race was on, especially because of the flu's impact on military readiness and strength. Military readiness, it seems, provided the crucial push for federal efforts to fund influenza vaccine development.[10]

Indeed, remembering the number of troops made "non-effective"[6] in World War I by influenza provided an impetus to quickly find a way to protect the troops sent to fight in World War II. While research on a flu vaccine was underway in the 1930s, progress accelerated during World War II. Clinical trials run by the US Army in 1943 proved that a vaccine made with inactivated virus and grown in chicken eggs was effective in preventing flu. With the US Army's support, these vaccines were developed by Drs. Thomas Francis Jr. and Jonas Salk, who served as lead researchers at the University of Michigan in the effort to develop the first inactivated flu vaccine.[11] The vaccine, effective against both the A and B strains of influenza, was used widely in 1944, particularly by American troops in Europe. The vaccine was then extended to civilian use in 1945.[12]

Another pioneer who contributed to flu vaccine research was Dr. Maurice Hilleman, who worked as chief of respiratory diseases at the Walter Reed Army Institute of Research in Washington, DC, in 1949. Hilleman would play a critical role in developing vaccines to address the second major flu pandemic. As recounted by renowned vaccine expert Dr. Paul Offit in his Hilleman biography, Hilleman anticipated a 1957 flu pandemic after reading an article in the newspaper. On the morning of April 17, 1957, he was sitting in his office at Walter Reed reading a *New York Times* article about an influenza outbreak in Hong Kong.[13,14] The article reported an estimated 250,000 people were infected, which was then about 10% of Hong Kong's population. The *Times* went on to report that tens of thousands of people lined up to receive health care, including "glassy-eyed" children. Hilleman put down the paper: "My God," he said, "this is the pandemic. It's here!"[13] Hilleman subsequently convinced reluctant US health officials to take notice and almost single-handedly shepherded a vaccine for use in the general public in just four months. Indeed, Hilleman's work may have been the first true Operation Warp Speed.

As a military doctor working at Walter Reed, Hilleman was able to quickly get samples of the virus from an infected US serviceman in Japan. After determining it to be a new flu virus for which people had little or no immunity, he coordinated with pharmaceutical companies to rapidly manufacture 40 million doses in time for the fall when children were to return to school. Hilleman's prediction turned out to be correct, and cases arrived on US shores that fall. Because of widespread availability of Hilleman's vaccine (the population of America was less than 180 million in 1957), the worst of the outbreak was averted and the new flu that could have claimed hundreds of thousands of victims was estimated to have 116,000 deaths in the United States.[13] According to the documentary film *Hilleman: A Perilous Quest to Save the World's Children,*[15] Hilleman's effort in 1957 was the first time one scientist had so significantly helped stop a pandemic in world history. Dr. Hilleman would go on to develop 9 of the 14 immunizations routinely administered to children today, making him the father of modern vaccines. He is also most likely one of the greatest scientists that most people have never heard of.[15]

In 1968, another flu pandemic emerged with first cases detected in Hong Kong in July of that year. The National Influenza Center at the University of Hong Kong isolated a new influenza A (H3N2) virus on July 17. The World Health Organization subsequently issued a global warning in August.[16] The first case in the United States was detected on September 2, 1968, in a soldier returning from the war in Vietnam. Even before cases were confirmed in America, the National Institute of Health's Division of Biologics Standards provided samples of the virus to vaccine manufacturers in August to start the vaccine development process. After initial adjustments, manufacturers released a first lot of 110,000 vaccine doses on November 15, 1968. An additional 15 million doses became available by the pandemic's peak in January 1969.[17] After the peak, vaccine demand waned despite an estimated 100,000 deaths. Unlike the response in 1957, Dr. Hilleman concluded in a review written for the World Health Organization that

> for the vast majority of persons in the USA, the new Hong Kong influenza vaccine was too little and too late. The amount of vaccine produced in time for use, in spite of heroic efforts, was far less than in the 1957 Asian influenza pandemic, when there was a 5-month warning

prior to the pandemic event, in contrast with the short 3-month warning of the Hong Kong influenza pandemic.[18]

The effect of the vaccine on reducing pandemic spread in 1968 was questionable as a result of the timing of its administration after the pandemic had already taken root, a theme to be repeated in the 2009 H1N1 pandemic.

THE SWINE FLU AFFAIR

In 1976, a significant incident took place in public health history that came to be known as the Swine Flu Affair. It began when a US Army recruit died of influenza at Fort Dix, New Jersey, in January 1976. Laboratory scientists from the Centers for Disease Control and Prevention (CDC) confirmed the case as a new flu strain traced to pigs. The novelty of the virus fired memories of the 1918–1919 pandemic and set off alarm bells across the federal government. According to an account written by Harvey Fineberg and Richard Neustadt, the government spent much of 1976 preparing a plan to vaccinate an unprecedented 213 million Americans.[19]

The resulting National Influenza Immunization Program, as it was formally named, was funded by a $135 million appropriation from Congress. The program was implemented by state health departments with support of grants and technical assistance from the federal Department of Health, Education, and Welfare (now Health and Human Services, or HHS). Vaccine administration started later in the outbreak than expected on October 1, 1976, with delays caused by difficulties in determining appropriate dosage for pediatric use and significant wrangling over liability coverage for vaccinators. In a national first, both President Jimmy Carter and First Lady Roslyn Carter were vaccinated on television to help boost confidence in the vaccine.

Within weeks, however, reports of a rare but serious side effect, Guillain-Barré syndrome, emerged. These reports raised questions about the vaccine's safety and began to erode the public's confidence in the new vaccine. On December 16, after 40 million vaccinations had occurred, the program was suspended to assess these adverse event reports. Among 40 million vaccinations, there were 532 cases of Guillain-Barré reported and 32 deaths.[20] Mass vaccinations never restarted, and in another unexpected twist, the swine flu never reappeared. In the aftermath of the entire affair, Dr. David Sencer, the CDC director at the time, was fired. The entire response was later characterized as a fiasco, and today the incident is held up to many students and decision makers as a case study of poor policy making.

In their famous after-action review entitled *The Swine Flu Affair: Decision-Making on a Slippery Disease*, authors Richard Neustadt and Harvey Fineberg identify seven leading features that influenced policy decision-making during the vaccination campaign. These include the following features[19(p1)]:

1. Overconfidence by specialists in theories spun from meager evidence.
2. Conviction fueled by a conjunction of some preexisting personal agendas.
3. Zeal by health professionals to make their lay superiors do right.
4. Premature commitment to deciding more than had to be decided.
5. Failure to address uncertainties in such a way as to prepare for reconsideration.
6. Insufficient questioning of scientific logic and of implementation prospects.
7. Insensitivity to media relations and the long-term credibility of institutions.

These factors pinpointed the difficulty in making policy with incomplete information and the impact of conflict and controversy. These issues would be ever present throughout the nation's COVID response almost half a century later. The controversy surrounding the Swine Flu Affair is a cautionary tale in the curriculum of most public health programs today.

TERRORISM AND PUBLIC HEALTH PREPAREDNESS

While these earlier influenza pandemics certainly informed contemporary pandemic planning, it was the terrorist attacks of September 11, 2001, and subsequent anthrax attacks weeks later that highlighted to the highest-level officials of the US government the need for improved public health preparedness and response. One week after planes hit the World Trade Center and the Pentagon, powdered anthrax spores were deliberately put into letters that were mailed through the US postal system. The letters infected 22 people, including 12 mail handlers, with anthrax, and 5 of them died. These anthrax attacks, while limited in scope, revealed our nation's lack of preparedness to deal with the deliberate release of a biological weapon. And because some of the letters were addressed to the Washington, DC, offices of several members of Congress, policymakers could not ignore the threat.

In the wake of these attacks, HHS created the Office of Public Health Emergency Preparedness in 2002. The goal of this office was to coordinate the preparedness and response functions of various federal agencies, including the CDC's nascent Bioterrorism Response Program located within the National Center for Infectious Diseases. The Office of Public Health Emergency Preparedness also provided initial funding to state, territorial, and local health departments and to hospitals and health care systems for bioterrorism planning. As a part of grant requirements, health departments and health systems were required to develop plans for receiving and distributing medical supplies, including vaccines, from the newly created CDC National Pharmaceutical Stockpile. Resources to support the bioterrorism planning effort came from $2.9 billion in emergency supplemental public health funding that was approved by Congress shortly after the attacks.[21] At the time, HHS noted this was nearly 10 times the $296 million to address bioterrorism that was available in 2001 before the attacks took place.[21]

It took almost three more years to secure additional funding for bioterrorism preparedness. In July 2004, Congress passed, and President George W. Bush signed, legislation called the Project BioShield Act to bolster additional funding for bioterrorism efforts and continue to support public health preparedness efforts. In remarks at the bill's signing, the president set the tone for a potentially distracting divide between funding for efforts to prepare for naturally occurring pathogens and preparedness for human-made bioterrorist threats, stating:

> On September the 11th, 2001, America saw the destruction and grief terrorists could inflict with commercial airlines turned into weapons of mass murder. Those attacks revealed the depth of our enemies' determination, but not the extent of their ambitions. We know that the terrorists seek an even deadlier technology. And if they acquire chemical, biological or nuclear weapons, we have no doubt they will use them to cause even greater harm. The bill I am about to sign is an important element in our response to that threat. By authorizing unprecedented funding and providing new capabilities, Project BioShield will help America purchase, develop and deploy cutting-edge defenses against catastrophic attack.[22]

The law included several provisions addressing the role of vaccine development in a potential bioterrorism attack. Most importantly, Project BioShield authorized $5.6 billion over 10 years for the US government to purchase and stockpile vaccines and drugs to fight anthrax, smallpox, and other potential bioterrorism agents.

At a ceremony in the White House Rose Garden, President Bush also announced that HHS had already taken steps to purchase 75 million doses of an improved anthrax vaccine for the nation's stockpile.[22] The president also highlighted the importance of strengthening a National Strategic Stockpile, originally called the National Pharmaceutical Stockpile, that had been created on a smaller scale in 1999.[23(p358)] He also confirmed how much the threat of a smallpox attack, not influenza pandemic, dominated preparedness planning in the wake of September 11, stating:

> Project BioShield is part of a broader strategy to defend America against the threat of weapons of mass destruction. Since September the 11th, we've increased funding for the Strategic National Stockpile by a factor of five, increased funding for biodefense research at NIH by a factor of 30, secured enough smallpox vaccine for every American, worked with cities on plans to deliver antibiotics and chemical antidotes in an emergency, improved the safety of our food supply, and deployed advanced environmental detectors under the BioWatch program to provide the earliest possible warning of a biological attack.[22]

Support for federal, state, and local plans to deliver medical countermeasures in an emergency fell to the division within CDC that had lead responsibility for administering the National Strategic Stockpile, which first issued guidance to state and local public health agencies for their plans shortly thereafter.

After a focus on the global war on terror and the threats of intentional bioterrorism, the focus of federal public health preparedness swung back to naturally occurring biological threats. President Bush was reported to have read an advance copy of John Barry's *The Great Influenza* while vacationing on his ranch in the summer of 2005. In the book, Barry tells the story of the 1918–1919 influenza pandemic and its grim devastation. Upon returning to Washington, DC, after his vacation, the president met with Fran Townsend, his national security advisor. He urgently told her, "You've got to read this . . . Look, this happens every 100 years. We need a national strategy," she later told ABC News.[24]

President Bush's realization of the threat that pandemic influenza could pose to the United States spurred the creation of the first national strategy for pandemic influenza, issued by the Homeland Security Council (HSC) as a 17-page document in November 2005.[25] The document's brevity caused some to call it "a plan to have a plan,"[26] but its core pillars established the fundamentals of national influenza preparedness planning. The HSC's *National Strategy* stated that the United States would develop a global early warning system for pandemic influenza; commit funding to develop new, rapid vaccine technology; and enhance the national stockpile with critical response supplies such as face masks and ventilators.

There was a clear focus on bolstering national capacity to quickly develop and manufacture vaccines to prevent pandemic flu, but just two bullet points in the entire original plan were devoted to the critical task of administering vaccines to the population:

Establishing Distribution Plans for Vaccines and Antivirals

It is essential that we prioritize the allocation of countermeasures (vaccines and antivirals) that are in limited supply and define effective distribution modalities during a pandemic. We will:

- Develop credible countermeasure distribution mechanisms for vaccine and antiviral agents prior to and during a pandemic
- Prioritize countermeasure allocation before an outbreak, and update this prioritization immediately after the outbreak begins based on the at-risk populations, available supplies and the characteristics of the virus.[25(pp5-6)]

Although thin on details, the HSC's *National Strategy* document indicated it would advance implementation plans and future guidance.

The HSC's *National Strategy for Pandemic Influenza* included a provision that would prove to be an Achilles heel in both the 2009 H1N1 pandemic response and during COVID. The strategy stated that the federal government would

work to ensure clear, effective and coordinated risk communication, domestically and internationally, before and during a pandemic. This includes identifying credible spokespersons at all levels of government to effectively coordinate and communicate helpful, informative messages in a timely manner.[25(p4)]

The widespread chaos experienced in the early weeks of COVID vaccine distribution may have been inevitable, but it was certainly hampered by a lack of consistent messaging on what the public should expect and who the government's credible spokespersons were. Similarly, the plan stressed the need to disseminate accurate, useful public health messages that should be tailored to local needs as needed and include information on the rationale for prioritization. Consistent, credible, and accurate messaging for use at the local level would be yet another challenge in the COVID response.

By the time the HSC's plan was distributed, some of the implementation planning was already underway within the CDC. Utilizing funding for public health preparedness appropriated to the CDC in the late 1990s, which was greatly increased with new funding authorized after the September 11 and anthrax attacks, the CDC had developed the Public Health Emergency Preparedness for Bioterrorism cooperative agreement program with state and territorial health departments and several large cities. Although CDC funds were intended to upgrade state and local public health jurisdictions' preparedness for and response to bioterrorism, outbreaks of other infectious diseases, and other public health threats and emergencies, they could also be used to support state efforts in conjunction with national response plans, including the HSC's *National Strategy*.[27]

In 2004, the CDC Public Health Emergency Preparedness for Bioterrorism program guidance introduced what was termed a measurement benchmark focused on public health preparedness for pandemic influenza. The guidance stated, "Its addition underscores the need to address current vulnerability to the emergence of an influenza strain—whether naturally occurring or terrorist-induced—for which humans have little or no protective immunity and for which an effective vaccine may not be available until the epidemic is far advanced or perhaps never."[27(p2)] The guidance directed states to "coordinate planning and program implementation activities to ensure that state and local health departments, hospitals, and other health care entities are able to mount a collective response"[27(p5)] to pandemic influenza that integrated public health laboratories, surveillance, communication, and other systems to work together. For the first time, states were directed to create jurisdictional plans for pandemic influenza.

In addition to the HSC's strategy, HHS released its *Pandemic Influenza Plan* in November 2005, calling it a "blueprint for all HHS pandemic influenza preparedness and response activities."[1(p8)] Heavily influenced by lessons learned from earlier influenza responses, including the pandemic of 1918–1919, the plan included the most detail to date on the planning assumptions to inform vaccine distribution in a pandemic event. One of eight "doctrines" introduced in the plan states, "At the onset of a pandemic, vaccine, which will initially be in short supply, will be procured by HHS and distributed to state and local health departments for immunization of predetermined priority groups."[1(p12)] The plan included a detailed nine-page discussion on work already completed to help state and local jurisdictions prioritize who should be first in line for a vaccine. It also directed states to fine-tune their own prioritization processes, stating:

Based on this guidance, state, local, and tribal implementation plans should be developed to (1) include more specific definitions of the priority groups (e.g., which functions are indeed critical to maintaining continuity) and their size; (2) define how persons in these groups will be identified; and (3) establish strategies for effectively and equitably delivering vaccines and antiviral drugs to these populations.[1(p60)]

In addition to the discussion of prioritization in the main guidance, the plan also included an appendix with even more detailed instructions for jurisdictions to plan for mass vaccine distribution.

One of the key points that would reemerge as a fundamental during COVID vaccine distribution was that the nation would build upon existing vaccine program infrastructure and channels of distribution already in place for seasonal flu vaccination. The HHS plan directed states and local health departments during the interpandemic period to work with health care partners to enhance levels of both seasonal influenza and pneumococcal vaccination in groups at risk for severe influenza and in health care workers. It noted:

> The success of the pandemic influenza vaccination program will be determined in large part by the strength of state and local vaccination programs during the Interpandemic Period. Higher annual vaccination rates will foster increased familiarity with vaccine distribution and public confidence in influenza vaccines, increased manufacturing capacity for influenza vaccines, and strengthened distribution channels.[1(pp276-277)]

The recommendations for "Interpandemic and Pandemic Alert Periods" focused on planning for vaccine distribution, vaccination of priority groups, monitoring of adverse events, tracking of vaccine supply and administration, vaccine coverage and effectiveness studies, communications, legal preparedness, and training.[1(p276)] The plan also provided a detailed list delineating the responsibilities of HHS and of state and local health departments both before and during pandemic vaccine distribution (included in an appendix at the end of this chapter). The list is notable because it spells out the essential activities that would be foundational to COVID vaccine distribution 15 years later. Unlike President Trump's Operation Warp Speed plans, however, the 2005 HHS document did not include any specified role for the US military.

Several policy pronouncements included in the 2005 HHS plan were either ignored or second-guessed when President Trump put the military in charge of the logistics of vaccine distribution during Operation Warp Speed. The 2005 plan stated that "distribution of pandemic vaccine to health departments and providers will occur via private-sector vaccine distributors or directly via manufacturer."[1(p278)] Our discussions with key officials with knowledge of Operation Warp Speed activities indicate that the program's officials were skeptical that the CDC's existing distributor would have the capacity to succeed. It took months for the CDC to convince them that reinventing this wheel was not warranted.

Other elements of federal pandemic influenza vaccine planning could have been included in model COVID vaccination plans had the previous influenza plans been consulted, with a few notable exceptions. The lead time to develop a flu vaccine matching the pandemic strain was expected to be four to six months, while with COVID, which is not an influenza virus and had never been seen before, the lead time was almost a full year. And while flu plans likely anticipated the need for two doses, which is the same for COVID, the prioritization of populations was markedly different because of the differing impact of the two diseases. While children were likely to be prioritized in pandemic influenza plans, children were less impacted with severe illness by COVID, and for the first several months of the COVID vaccination campaign, there was no authorized vaccine for individuals under age 18.

In May 2006, the HSC issued a 233-page *National Strategy for Pandemic Influenza Implementation Plan,*[28] as a follow-on to the 17-page *National Strategy* it released in 2005. The *Implementation Plan* includes extensive discussion of improving the capacity and speed for manufacturing flu vaccine but is notably light on vaccine distribution planning details, offering only the following two references:

> 6.1.13. Develop credible countermeasure distribution mechanisms for vaccine and antiviral agents prior to and during a pandemic.
>> 6.1.13.1. HHS, in coordination with DHS, DOD, VA, and DOJ, and in collaboration with State, local, and tribal partners and the private sector, shall ensure that States, localities, and tribal entities have developed and exercised pandemic influenza countermeasure distribution plans, and can enact security protocols if necessary, according to pre-determined priorities . . . within 12 months. Measures of performance: ability to activate, deploy, and begin distributing contents of medical stockpiles in localities as needed established and validated through exercises.[28(p122)]
>
> 6.3.5.3. HHS, in coordination with DHS, shall allocate and assure the effective and secure distribution of public stocks of antiviral drugs and vaccines when they become available. HHS and DHS are currently prepared to distribute stockpile as soon as countermeasures become available. Measure of performance: number of doses of vaccine and treatment courses of antiviral medications distributed.[28(p142)]

Because they played critical roles in its development, CDC officials were familiar with all these pandemic influenza plans. Even though Trump-appointed officials would later claim that no planning had occurred before their arrival, the pandemic influenza plans provided a solid foundation that was eventually used to plan for COVID vaccine distribution.[29]

A PRECURSOR TO COVID: THE 2009 H1N1 INFLUENZA PANDEMIC

In April 2009, less than three years after issuing the *Implementation Plan*, a new influenza virus emerged, causing the first pandemic in over 40 years and providing a real-world chance to apply these newly developed plans. Within one week of virus detection, the CDC was working on vaccine candidates.[30] On April 26, the US government declared the 2009 H1N1 flu a public health emergency of international concern. Just several days later, in a move foreshadowing widespread school closures due to COVID, the CDC issued its *School (K–12) Dismissal and Childcare Facilities: Interim CDC Guidance in Response to Human Infections with the Influenza A H1N1 Virus.*[31] In the guidance, the agency recommended a seven-day dismissal in schools and childcare facilities with laboratory-confirmed cases of influenza A (H1N1) virus. On June 11, 2009, the World Health Organization declared H1N1 a pandemic reflecting the virus's spread to other parts of the world.[30]

During the summer of 2009, HHS told states, localities, and the public to expect that more than 100 million doses of the H1N1 vaccine would be available by October. After some drop-off in cases over the summer of 2009, a second wave of infections began in August while vaccine trials were already underway. On September 15, the Food and Drug Administration (FDA) announced the approval of four flu vaccines, just five months after the new virus strain was first identified.

The CDC's previous pandemic planning had focused on direct vaccine distribution by manufacturers to a limited number of sites designated by state and territorial health departments. But according to a subsequent report by the Government Accountability Office (GAO), officials had decided that using a private distributor that routinely distributes seasonal influenza and other vaccines to existing clinical settings was a preferable method because of the efficiencies of using an existing system and scaling it.[32] This decision built upon the centralized distributor system utilized in the CDC's successful Vaccines for Children (VFC) program. In 2009, the VFC program's central distributor shipped the H1N1 vaccine from regional distribution centers that received the H1N1 vaccines from five vaccine manufacturers to individual providers and organizations identified by state and local jurisdictions. State and local health officials, in conjunction with professional associations such as the American Medical Association, identified providers who signed agreements to administer the H1N1 vaccine, including providers who had not previously participated in the VFC program, such as obstetricians, gynecologists, and other physicians who treat and immunize adults, to expand the pool of health professionals who could vaccinate.

States began ordering vaccine by the end of September 2009, and the first shots were given on October 5. But by the end of October, less than 17 million doses of the promised 100 million had been shipped due to production issues. Finally, by late December, more than 100 million doses of vaccine became available; after initial targeting to the most high-risk groups (pregnant women, children and young adults age 6 months to 24 years, and adults age 25 to 64 who had health conditions that put them at high risk of medical complications from influenza), vaccine eligibility opened to anyone who wanted it. However, by that point in the outbreak, the peak of flu activity had passed and demand for the vaccine softened as most of the public lost interest in being vaccinated.

Nevertheless, by January 2010, approximately 124 million doses of 2009 H1N1 vaccine had been distributed, and the CDC estimated 81 million doses had been administered.[33] By August, the WHO declared the H1N1 pandemic over. In the United States, the 2009 outbreak turned out to be as or less severe than seasonal influenza outbreaks, with an estimated 12,469 deaths,[34] compared to the 12,000 to 52,000 deaths annually from seasonal flu estimated by the CDC.[35]

According to a 2011 GAO study of the lessons learned from H1N1, "When reality didn't meet the public expectations set by HHS, government credibility took a hit. State and local health departments had to cancel planned vaccination clinics and change their public messaging when the H1N1 vaccine wasn't available when expected."[36] In a key finding that would later play out during COVID, the GAO review further illuminated this key lesson from the H1N1 response:

> Effective communication on the availability of vaccine is central to a successful response. Although the federal government was able to purchase and distribute millions of doses of H1N1 vaccine, the vaccine was not widely available when the public expected it and at the peak of demand. Because the failure to effectively manage public expectations can undermine government credibility, it is essential that vaccine production efforts be paired with effective communication strategies regarding the availability of the vaccine.[32(p44)]

PRE-COVID CDC AND STATE LEADERSHIP IN VACCINE DISTRIBUTION

The H1N1 pandemic of 2009 relied on vaccine delivery infrastructure supported by the CDC's VFC program created by Congress in 1993. However, the roots of the CDC's unrivaled leadership in vaccine distribution go back over 50 years to when Congress passed the Vaccination Assistance Act of 1962 to assist US jurisdictions in purchasing vaccine doses for polio, diphtheria, pertussis, tetanus, and measles, which was added in 1965, creating the Section 317 Immunization Program.[37] Together, the CDC's Section 317 Program and VFC program are credited with achieving record high vaccination rates among America's children. They have been so effective in eliminating infectious diseases that many of the nation's pediatricians practicing today have never or rarely seen diseases that were once common killers of scores of children in the era before widespread vaccine administration.

The Section 317 Program receives an annual appropriation by the US Congress to provide support for a range of critical activities and provide a safety net for those who cannot otherwise access immunization services. The program provides grants to 64 US jurisdictions, including all 50 states, the District of Columbia, 5 large cities, 5 US territories, and 3 Pacific freely associated states. These grants are used to support the immunization workforce at the state and local levels to recruit and educate networks of immunization providers, provide continual quality assurance, promote public awareness of new and expanded vaccine recommendations, manage vaccine shortages, and prepare for and respond to vaccine-preventable outbreaks.[38] Other activities support direct public vaccine provision; oversee provider quality by conducting assessments, training programs, and compliance monitoring; develop immunization registries; support school-based and community-based service delivery programs; create and deliver consumer information; conduct vaccine-preventable disease surveillance; and conduct population needs assessments. Grants are also used by jurisdictions to monitor the safety and effectiveness of vaccines and vaccine programs.[39(p57)]

Each jurisdiction's program is led by an immunization program manager who provides overall leadership and accountability for all immunization activities in their state or locality. These individuals come to the role from a variety of backgrounds, including former Peace Corps volunteers, Jesuit Volunteer Corps alums, labor and delivery nurses, sexually transmitted infection control, epidemiology, medicine, and a range of other fields. What they all have in common is a dedication to eliminating vaccine preventable disease. While only a few of the immunization program leaders responding to COVID were in their roles in 2009, all were familiar with their jurisdiction's pandemic influenza vaccine planning. All stood ready to build upon those plans when the COVID pandemic began, but at the same time they were keenly aware of the gaps in the nation's immunization infrastructure, particularly in state systems serving adults.

A major reason for gaps in the immunization infrastructure is that while the Section 317 Program provides critical funding to all states and some local jurisdictions, the funding levels provided by Congress have never met the identified needs. An annual assessment conducted by experts at the CDC and presented to Congress in what is known as a professional judgment budget has consistently identified a gap of close to $800 million between extant funding and needed funding and has recommended that $1.4 billion is required to meet the nation's immunization program needs.[40] Instead, in the most recent year for which information is available, the total program funding level was $651 million, of which about $340 million was provided to states and other eligible jurisdictions, with the remaining funds supporting essential activities at the CDC.[41(p76)] Funding levels for the program were stagnant for most of the decade preceding the emergence of COVID.

The CDC Immunization Services Division works with 64 Section 317-funded jurisdictions that deliver about 75 million doses of routine childhood vaccines through VFC every year.[42] The CDC also works with these jurisdictions to prepare and deliver flu vaccine campaigns on an annual basis and to prepare for the possibility of a flu pandemic. As noted, when the H1N1 flu pandemic hit in 2009, HHS utilized this existing vaccine purchase and distribution system created by VFC to rapidly deliver vaccines nationwide.

Significant federal resources have gone into planning for pandemic influenza preparedness and response in the years since the 2001 terrorist attacks. In addition, earlier pandemics have not only proved that the nation's public health agencies have the capacity to respond to pandemics but also identified areas for continued improvement. While COVID is not influenza, many of the assumptions of influenza planning guided state and federal thinking in the early months of the pandemic. The next two chapters examine how the Trump administration's approach diverged from existing federal plans and initially discounted the role of public health agencies in favor of the private sector as they planned for the most complex public health campaign in American history.

REFERENCES

1. US Department of Health and Human Services. HHS pandemic influenza plan. November 2005. Available at: https://www.cdc.gov/flu/pandemic-resources/pdf/hhspandemicinfluenzaplan.pdf. Accessed September 10, 2022.

2. Mak T. Weeks before virus panic, Intelligence chairman privately raised alarm, sold stocks. *Morning Edition*. National Public Radio. March 19, 2020. Available at: https://www.npr.org/2020/03/19/818192535/burr-recording-sparks-questions-about-private-comments-on-covid-19. Accessed September 10, 2022.

3. Last JM. *A Dictionary of Epidemiology*. 4th ed. New York, NY: Oxford University Press; 2021.

4. Centers for Disease Control and Prevention. Past pandemics. August 10, 2018. Available at: https://www.cdc.gov/flu/pandemic-resources/basics/past-pandemics.html. Accessed September 10, 2022.

5. MPH Online. Outbreak: 10 of the worst pandemics in history. August 31, 2021. Available at: https://www.mphonline.org/worst-pandemics-in-history. Accessed September 10, 2022.

6. Byerly CR. (2010). The US military and the influenza pandemic of 1918–1919. *Public Health Rep*. 2010;125(suppl 3):82–91.

7. Dutton LK, Rhee PC, Shin AY, Ehrlichman RJ, Shemin RJ. (2021). Combating an invisible enemy: the American military response to global pandemics. *Military Med Res*. 2021;8(1). https://doi.org/10.1186/s40779-021-00299-3.

8. Barry JM. *The Great Influenza: The Story of the Deadliest Pandemic in History*. New York, NY: Penguin Books; 2020.

9. Najera R. The 1918–19 Spanish influenza pandemic and vaccine development. History of Vaccines. September 26, 2018. Available at: https://historyofvaccines.org/blog/the-1918-19-spanish-influenza-pandemic-and-vaccine-development. Accessed September 10, 2022.

10. Francis T. The development of the 1943 vaccination, study of the Commission on Influenza. *Am J Hyg*. 1945;42(1):1–11.

11. Centers for Disease Control and Prevention. Influenza historic timeline. January 30, 2019. Available at: https://www.cdc.gov/flu/pandemic-resources/pandemic-timeline-1930-and-beyond.htm. Accessed September 10, 2022.

12. Hannoun C. The evolving history of influenza viruses and influenza vaccines. *Medscape.* November 12, 2013. Available at: https://www.medscape.com/viewarticle/812621_3. Accessed September 10, 2022.

13. Offit PA. *Vaccinated: One Man's Quest to Defeat the World's Deadliest Diseases.* New York, NY: Harper Perennial; 2008.

14. Hong Kong battling influenza epidemic. *New York Times.* April 17, 1957. Available at: https://www.nytimes.com/1957/04/17/archives/hong-kong-battling-influenza-epidemic.html. Accessed September 10, 2022.

15. Children's Hospital of Philadelphia. Hilleman: A Perilous Quest to Save the World's Children. 2016. Available at: https://hillemanfilm.com. Accessed September 10, 2022.

16. Jester BJ, Uyeki TM, Jernigan DB. Fifty years of influenza A(H3N2) following the pandemic of 1968. *Am J Public Health.* 2020;110(5):669–676. doi:10.2105/ajph.2019.305557.

17. Murray R. Production and testing in the USA of influenza virus vaccine made from the Hong Kong variant in 1968–69. *Bull World Health Organ.* 1969;41(3–4–5):493–496.

18. Hilleman MR. The roles of early alert and of adjuvant in the control of Hong Kong influenza by vaccines. *Bull World Health Organ.* 1969;41(3):623–628.

19. Neustadt RE, Fineberg HV. *The Swine Flu Affair: Decision-Making on a Slippery Disease.* Honolulu, HI: University Press of the Pacific; 2005.

20. Saunders-Hastings P, Krewski D. Reviewing the history of pandemic influenza: understanding patterns of emergence and transmission. *Pathogens.* 2016;5(4):66. doi:10.3390/pathogens5040066.

21. CIDRAP. HHS to release $200 million in bioterrorism preparedness funds to states. January 28, 2002. Available at: https://www.cidrap.umn.edu/news-perspective/2002/01/hhs-release-200-million-bioterrorism-preparedness-funds-states. Accessed September 10, 2022.

22. National Archives and Records Administration. Remarks by the president at the signing of S.15—Project Bioshield Act of 2004. July 21, 2004. Available at: https://georgewbush-whitehouse.archives.gov/news/releases/2004/07/20040721-2.html. Accessed September 10, 2022.

23. Omnibus Consolidated and Emergency Supplemental Appropriations Act of 1999, HR 4328, 105th Cong, (1998). Available at: https://www.congress.gov/105/plaws/publ277/PLAW-105publ277.pdf. Accessed September 10, 2022.

24. Mosk M. George W. Bush in 2005: "If we wait for a pandemic to appear, it will be too late to prepare." *ABC News.* April 5, 2020. Available at: https://abcnews.go.com/Politics/george-bush-2005-wait-pandemic-late-prepare/story?id=69979013. Accessed September 24, 2022.

25. Homeland Security Council. National strategy for pandemic influenza. November 2005. Available at: https://www.cdc.gov/flu/pandemic-resources/pdf/pandemic-influenza-strategy-2005.pdf. Accessed September 10, 2022.

26. Lewis M. *The Premonition: A Pandemic Story.* New York, NY: W. W. Norton & Company; 2021.

27. Centers for Disease Control and Prevention. Continuation guidance for cooperative agreement on public health preparedness and response for bioterrorism. June 14, 2004. Available at: https://www.cdc.gov/cpr/documents/coopagreement-archive/fy2004/guidance_intro.pdf. Accessed September 23, 2022.

28. Homeland Security Council. National strategy for pandemic influenza: implementation plan. May 2006. Available at: https://www.cdc.gov/flu/pandemic-resources/pdf/pandemic-influenza-implementation.pdf. Accessed September 10, 2022.

29. Martin D. Operation Warp Speed: planning the distribution of a future COVID-19 vaccine. *CBS News.* November 9, 2020. Available at: https://www.cbsnews.com/video/covid-19-vaccine-distribution-60-minutes-2020-11-08. Accessed September 10, 2022.

30. Centers for Disease Control and Prevention. 2009 H1N1 pandemic timeline. May 8, 2019. Available at: https://www.cdc.gov/flu/pandemic-resources/2009-pandemic-timeline.html. Accessed September 10, 2022.

31. Centers for Disease Control and Prevention. CDC health update: school (K-12) dismissal and childcare facilities: interim CDC guidance in response to human infections with the influenza A H1N1 virus. May 1, 2009. Available at: https://www.cdc.gov/h1n1flu/HAN/050109.htm. Accessed September 10, 2022.

32. US Government Accountability Office. Influenza pandemic: lessons from the H1N1 pandemic should be incorporated into future planning. June 27, 2011. Available at: https://www.gao.gov/products/gao-11-632. Accessed September 11, 2022.

33. Centers for Disease Control and Prevention. Final estimates for 2009–10 seasonal influenza and influenza A (H1N1) 2009 monovalent vaccination coverage—United States, August 2009 through May 2010. May 13, 2011. Available at: https://www.cdc.gov/flu/fluvaxview/coverage_0910estimates.htm. Accessed September 11, 2022.

34. Centers for Disease Control and Prevention. 2009 H1N1 pandemic. June 11, 2019. Available at: https://www.cdc.gov/flu/pandemic-resources/2009-h1n1-pandemic.html. Accessed September 11, 2022.

35. Centers for Disease Control and Prevention. Frequently asked questions about estimated flu burden. October 21, 2021. Available at: https://www.cdc.gov/flu/about/burden/faq.htm. Accessed September 11, 2022.

36. US Government Accountability Office. COVID-19 vaccines and the lessons learned from H1N1. January 14, 2021. Available at: https://www.gao.gov/blog/covid-19-vaccines-and-lessons-learned-h1n1. Accessed September 11, 2022.

37. Rein DB, Honeycutt AA, Rojas-Smith L, Hersey JC. Impact of the CDC's Section 317 Immunization Grants Program funding on childhood vaccination coverage. *Am J Public Health.* 2006;96(9):1548–1553. doi:10.2105/ajph.2005.078451.

38. National Vaccine Advisory Committee. Protecting the public's health: critical functions of the Section 317 Immunization Program—a report of the National Vaccine Advisory Committee. *Public Health Rep.* 2013;128:78–95. doi:10.1177/003335491312800203.

39. US Department of Health and Human Services, Centers for Disease Control and Prevention. Justification of estimates for appropriation committees. Available at: https://www.cdc.gov/budget/documents/fy2020/fy-2020-cdc-congressional-justification.pdf. Accessed September 11, 2022.

40. US Department of Health and Human Services, Centers for Disease Control and Prevention. Report to Congress on Section 317 Immunization Program—cost estimates. April 2021. Available at: https://www.317coalition.org/_files/ugd/cbc5b5_1189e28de678412a8349f977b05d9ab4.pdf. Accessed September 11, 2022.

41. US Department of Health and Human Services, Centers for Disease Control and Prevention. Justification of estimates for appropriation committees. Available at: https://www.cdc.gov/budget/documents/fy2023/FY-2023-CDC-congressional-justification.pdf. Accessed September 11, 2022.

42. Centers for Disease Control and Prevention, National Center for Immunization and Respiratory Diseases. Pandemic vaccine program: distribution, tracking, administration, and monitoring. 2020. Available at: https://www.cdc.gov/flu/pdf/pandemic-resources/pandemic-influenza-vaccine-distribution-9p-508.pdf. Accessed September 11, 2022.

Appendix 2A

Many of the roles and responsibilities for distribution of vaccine by the public health system were written into federal plans in 2005 and 2006.[1,2,3] The military and political officials President Trump placed in charge of vaccine distribution initially discounted the role of public health agencies in favor of private-sector partners and consequently diverted from these plans. The roles initially envisioned for public health in the 2005 HHS *Pandemic Influenza Plan* are included below as an example.[1(pp274-275)]

SUMMARY OF PUBLIC HEALTH ROLES AND RESPONSIBILITIES FOR VACCINE DISTRIBUTION AND USE

Interpandemic and Pandemic Alert Periods

State and local health departments:

- Work with health care partners and other stakeholders to develop state-based plans for vaccine effectiveness, safety, distribution, and use.

HHS agencies:

- Work with manufacturers to expedite public-sector vaccine purchasing contracts during a pandemic.
- Establish mechanisms for vaccine procurement and distribution.
- Develop guidance on priority groups for vaccination.
- Develop and stockpile vaccine for influenza strains with pandemic potential.
- Expedite the rapid development, licensure, and production of new influenza vaccines, as well as evaluate dose optimization strategies to maximize use of limited vaccine stocks.
- Estimate rates of reports of mild and severe adverse events following immunization (AEFIs) that may occur with mass influenza vaccination, and improve capacity for responding to them.
- Identify mechanisms and define protocols for conducting vaccine-effectiveness studies.
- Develop a system for monitoring state-specific vaccine coverage rates at regular intervals, using a preexisting population-based survey.

- Develop reporting specifications for tracking data on vaccine administration and provide a vaccine database for optional use by states.
- Develop and distribute communication and education materials for use by states and other stakeholders.

Pandemic Period

After the first reports of pandemic influenza are confirmed and before a pandemic vaccine becomes available

State and local health departments:

- If stockpiled vaccine of the pandemic subtype is available, work with health care partners and other stakeholders to distribute, deliver, and administer vaccines to designated groups.
- Mobilize health care partners, and prepare to activate state-based plans for distributing and administering vaccines.
- Keep the health care and public health workforce up to date on projected timelines for availability of vaccines against pandemic influenza.
- Review modifications, if any, to recommendations on vaccinating priority groups.
- Accelerate training in vaccination and vaccine monitoring for public health staff and for partners responsible for vaccinating priority groups.
- Work with other governmental agencies and nongovernmental organizations to ensure effective public health communications.

HHS agencies:

- Facilitate vaccine procurement, distribution, and tracking, working with private partners.
- Revise recommendations on vaccination of priority groups, guided by epidemiologic information about the pandemic virus (e.g., virulence, transmissibility, drug resistance, geographic spread, age-specific attack rates, morbidity and mortality rates).
- Provide state and local partners with guidance on reporting specifications for tracking administration of vaccine doses, to be used when vaccine becomes available.
- Provide state and local partners with guidance on Investigational New Drug (IND) and Emergency Use Authorization (EUA) procedures if new types of influenza vaccines for pandemic purposes are developed but not yet FDA approved.
- Provide guidance to state and local health departments on which adverse event reports are highest priority for investigation.
- Provide regulatory guidance to vaccine manufacturers for the manufacture and shipment of pandemic vaccines.

After a vaccine becomes available

State and local health departments:

- Work with health care partners and other stakeholders to distribute, deliver, and administer pandemic vaccines to priority groups.
- Monitor vaccine supplies, distribution, and use.
- Monitor and investigate adverse events.
- Phase-in vaccination of the rest of the population after priority groups have been vaccinated.
- Provide updated information to the public via the news media.
- Work with federal partners to evaluate vaccine-related response activities when the pandemic is over.

HHS agencies:

- Provide forecasts of pandemic vaccine availability from manufacturers.
- Continue to provide input into appropriate strain selection for seasonal influenza vaccine.
- Distribute public stocks of vaccines to state and large city health departments and to federal agencies with direct patient care responsibility, as needed.
- Implement protocols for assessing vaccine effectiveness.
- Monitor vaccine coverage rates.

REFERENCES

1. US Department of Health and Human Services. HHS pandemic influenza plan. November 2005. Available at: https://www.cdc.gov/flu/pandemic-resources/pdf/hhspandemicinfluenzaplan.pdf. Accessed September 10, 2022.
2. Homeland Security Council. National strategy for pandemic influenza. November 2005. Available at: https://www.cdc.gov/flu/pandemic-resources/pdf/pandemic-influenza-strategy-2005.pdf. Accessed September 10, 2022.
3. Homeland Security Council. National strategy for pandemic influenza: implementation plan. May 2006. Available at: https://www.cdc.gov/flu/pandemic-resources/pdf/pandemic-influenza-implementation.pdf. Accessed September 10, 2022.

3

Moving at Warp Speed

Today I want to update you on the next stage of this momentous medical initiative. It's called Operation Warp Speed. That means big, and it means fast . . . Its objective is to finish developing and then to manufacture and distribute a proven coronavirus vaccine as fast as possible . . . The great national project will bring together the best of American industry and innovation, the full resources of the United States Government, and the excellence and precision of the United States military. We have the military totally involved.[1]

–President Donald Trump, Remarks at the kickoff of Operation Warp Speed, Rose Garden, May 15, 2020

The deep state, or whoever, over at the FDA is making it very difficult for drug companies to get people in order to test the vaccines and therapeutics. Obviously, they are hoping to delay the answer until after November 3rd. Must focus on speed, and saving lives![2]

–President Donald Trump, August 22, 2020

The historically rapid development of COVID vaccines is a modern medical marvel that should have been one of President Trump's greatest achievements. Leading an effort to develop, manufacture, and begin distribution of a new vaccine for a novel virus in less than a year was unprecedented and was considered improbable. Most experts, including Dr. Anthony Fauci, didn't think it could be done.[3] The superlatives used to describe the Trump administration's plan strained adjectives and stretched clichés, but to many that did not matter: we were going all in on developing a COVID vaccine. Indeed, the attempt was called the biggest effort since the Manhattan Project that ended World War II. Operation Warp Speed (OWS), as the project would be known, would be the greatest logistical challenge in American history and potentially the greatest public health campaign of any generation.

"President Trump's vision for a vaccine by January 2021 will be one of the greatest scientific and humanitarian accomplishments in history," said Health and Human Services (HHS) secretary Alex Azar on the day it was announced.[1] And while a safe and effective vaccine was developed, manufactured, and delivered in record time under Donald Trump's watch, the seeds that undermined his achievement were planted well before he launched the warp speed effort.

President Trump's insistence on speed while simultaneously downplaying the seriousness of the virus broke all the rules of crisis communication. Even as he announced the drive to develop a vaccine, he expressed confidence the coronavirus would go away with or without a vaccine, stating at the Rose Garden ceremony, "And I just want to make something clear. It's very important: Vaccine or no vaccine, we're back. And we're starting the process. And in many cases, they don't have vaccines, and a virus or a flu comes, and you fight through it. We haven't seen anything like this in 100-and-some-odd years—1917."[1]

These mixed messages directly contributed to the further politicization of the pandemic response by minimizing the severity of the virus, which led the president's supporters to trivialize it while simultaneously investing billions to stop it. President Trump later undermined faith in the Food and Drug Administration (FDA), the nation's preeminent regulatory agency that would be called on to ensure the vaccine was safe and effective. He sidelined the Centers for Disease Control and Prevention (CDC) as "ineffective" and a "waste of time,"[4] but the agency would play a leading role in working with states and pharmacies to distribute vaccines. And by placing military leaders with virtually no experience in public health or vaccine development in command of its distribution, he introduced delay, duplication, and uncertainty into an enterprise that the CDC and HHS planners had been effectively carrying out for decades.

LAUNCHING OPERATION WARP SPEED

Operation Warp Speed was introduced on an unseasonably hot day on May 15, 2020. President Donald Trump took the podium in the White House Rose Garden surrounded by health officials from HHS and others from the Department of Defense (DoD). Notably absent were any leading officials from the CDC who had decades of experience in delivering tens of millions of vaccines across every community in America. The president's entourage did, however, include his secretary of defense Mark Esper and a four-star army general, Gustave Perna, who was taking over as the lead in distributing a biological product he admittedly knew very little about.

The president took the podium and began with some small talk about the hot weather. Moving to his script, he acknowledged the officials surrounding him. "Today I want to update you on the next stage of this momentous medical initiative. It's called Operation Warp Speed,"[1] the president announced, before adding his standard superlatives:

> That means big and it means fast—a massive scientific, industrial and logistical endeavor unlike anything our country has seen since the Manhattan Project. You really could say that nobody's seen anything like we're doing, whether it's ventilators or testing. Nobody's seen anything like we're doing now within our country since the Second World War. Incredible.[1]

And then he announced both the goal and a time frame that inadvertently fanned the flames of vaccine hesitancy: "Its objective is to finish developing and then to manufacture and distribute a proven coronavirus vaccine as fast as possible. Again, we'd love to see if we could do it prior to the end of the year. We think we're going to have some very good results coming out very quickly."[1]

Notably, the stress was on speed, with virtually no discussion of the FDA-led process to test and ensure safety. In fact, the president's full statement that day included 15 references to "speed," 10 uses of the word "quickly," 4 references to "fast," and only a passing reference to safety, and that was in the context of providing federal resources, "to safely expedite the trials."[1] As concerning as the focus on speed was to many, the introduction of the military into the domestic vaccine distribution process, which was previously the domain of the CDC and state health departments in conjunction with private-sector partners, may have been even more jolting to public health professionals. The president continued:

> The great national project will bring together the best of American industry and innovation, the full resources of the United States government, and the excellence and precision of the United States military. We have the military totally involved . . . This historic partnership will now bring together the full resources of the Department of Health and Human Services with the Department of Defense. And we know what that means. That means the full power and strength of military—the military. And that—really, talking about the logistics—if we get it, when we get it. That means the logistics, getting it out, so that everybody can take it.[1]

To be sure, many understood that bringing the military's contracting logistics to the project was necessary and made sense, given the scale required of a comprehensive COVID vaccine distribution process. Warlike effort was required in fighting the COVID scourge, and the government administration had the ability to invoke the Defense Production Act to force the prioritization of certain raw materials and expedite the supply chain when necessary. Perhaps most important, the ability to quickly expand urgently needed manufacturing capacity was recognized as beyond the immediate capacity of HHS. It made sense to engage DoD expertise in manufacturing and procurement.

But for decades the CDC and state health agencies had successfully operated as a public-private system that utilized a private-sector commercial vaccine distributor. This system had been used to distribute 75 million doses of vaccine annually,[5] and it had scaled up to deliver over 80 million doses of flu vaccine during the 2009 H1N1 pandemic.[6] It would certainly need to be expanded to meet the challenge of COVID, but what the president was announcing in the Rose Garden set off alarm bells among some public health officials: it seemed the administration was proposing to create a new, untested, and potentially duplicative system for COVID vaccine distribution. Furthermore, the president's proclamation that the military was "totally involved"[1] was imprecise enough a statement to raise the potential that Americans might see uniformed soldiers administering the vaccine. While the National Guard is often a welcome and necessary component of the response to emergencies, delicate questions were raised about whether US Army troops would be trusted vaccinators in certain communities.

President Trump then moved to introduce the OWS leadership:

> Today, we're proud to announce the addition of two of the most highly respected and skilled professionals in our country—worldwide respected. Operation Warp Speed's chief scientist will be Dr. Moncef Slaoui, a world-renowned immunologist who helped create 14 new vaccines—that's a lot of our new vaccines—in 10 years, during his time in the private sector. One of the most respected men in the world in the production and, really, on the formulation of vaccines.
>
> Joining Dr. Slaoui as Chief Operating Officer will be General Gus Perna, a four-star general who currently oversees 190,000 service members, civilians, and contractors as Commander of the US Army Materiel Command. That means logistics. That means getting it out. We got to get it out there.[1]

The president then made his first mention of the massive federal investment that would be attached to this effort. He stressed again the focus on speed, and he introduced the idea that vaccine development, manufacturing, and distribution were intertwined and essentially moving on parallel tracks. "Through Operation Warp Speed," he said, "the federal government is providing unprecedented support and resources to safely expedite the trials, moving on at record, record, record speed. While we accelerate the final phases of vaccine trials, Operation Warp Speed will be simultaneously accelerating its manufacturing and manufacturing process."[1]

Alluding to how moving forward with manufacturing vaccine before it was proven safe and effective would be one of the keys to saving time, the president said: "In other words, we're getting ready so that when we get the good word—that we have the vaccine, we have the formula, we have what we need—we're ready to go, as opposed to taking years to gear up. We're gearing up. It's risky, it's expensive, but we'll be saving massive amounts of time."[1] The president then underscored how the urgency of the pandemic justified this risky and expensive approach:

> Typically pharmaceutical companies wait to manufacture a vaccine—a vaccine until it has received all of the regulatory approvals necessary, and this can delay vaccines' availability to the public as much as a year and even more than that. However, our task is so urgent that, under Operation Warp Speed, the federal government will invest in manufacturing all of the top vaccine candidates before they're approved. So we're knowing exactly what we're doing before they're approved. That means they better come up with a good vaccine, because we're ready to deliver it.
>
> This will eliminate any unnecessary delay and enable us to begin providing Americans with a proven vaccine the day our scientists say, "We're ready, we got it."[1]

After the president's formal remarks, he turned to introduce the two men he tapped to colead the effort. General Perna then took the podium. "Thank you for this great honor for allowing me to be a part of this team," the general began. "It is going to be a Herculean task," he later acknowledged, "but the combination of the two main partners—between Health and Human Services and the Department of Defense—their combined strengths, partnered with the other teammates, will ensure our success."[1]

The general then highlighted the logistical capabilities of the military, omitting any reference to the existing capacity at CDC or in state and local health departments to deliver and administer vaccines. "One of the great advantages that we have as a military is our ability to do logistical and sustainment operations afar. We're just going to apply those capabilities to this mission. This mission is about defeating the enemy. We will defeat the enemy."[1] It was the first indication that the military leadership thought that delivering a completely novel biological product that needs to be injected into human beings would be the same as delivering supplies to the battlefield.

After remarks by General Perna, Dr. Slaoui, and Secretary of Defense Mark Esper, President Trump took questions from the press. Even though most public health experts were convinced that a safe and effective vaccine would be the best path to ending the pandemic, the president seemed to undermine even the need for a vaccine and once again could not resist the opportunity to minimize the danger posed by COVID. Picking up on a comment the president made in response to an earlier question, when a reporter asked, "Mr. President, you said, 'No vaccine . . .'—'Vaccine or no vaccine, we're back.' What did you mean by that?" The president responded:

> We think we're going to have a vaccine in the pretty near future. And if we do, we're going to really be a big step ahead. And if we don't, we're going to be like so many other cases, where you had a problem come in, it'll go away—at some point, it'll go away. It may flare up, and it may not flare up. We'll have to see what happens. But if it does flare up, we're going to put out the fire and we'll put it out quickly and efficiently. We've learned a lot.

When the next reporter asked the president how he thought the administration could develop vaccines faster than projected, he again discounted the very vaccine project he was announcing by saying:

> … But again, it's not solely vaccine based. Other things have never had a vaccine and they go away. I don't want people to think that this is all dependent on a vaccine, but a vaccine would be a tremendous thing.[1]

In his opening speech, President Trump had again stressed speed over safety, stating: "Another essential pillar of our strategy to keep America open is the development of effective treatments and vaccines as quickly as possible. Want to see if we can do that very quickly. We're looking to—when I say 'quickly,' we're looking to get it by the end of the year if we can. Maybe before."[1] It was the first public indication that the president was hoping to have a vaccine approved before the upcoming presidential election on

November 3. It was an acknowledgment that the vaccine development enterprise was happening against the backdrop of a bitterly contested national election.

The president offered another answer to another question that would not wear well over time. Asked, "Would a US vaccine be available for the rest of the world at an affordable rate?" he responded, "The last thing anybody is looking for is profit in terms of what we're doing. Every company, they want to get it out."[1] As of this writing, Pfizer reported nearly $37 billion in COVID vaccines sales for 2021, contributing to $22 billion in overall profits last year, making it "one of the most lucrative products in history."[7] Moderna posted revenue of $18.5 billion for the year 2021, nearly all of it from COVID-19 vaccine sales.[8] Both companies predict continued strong growth for COVID vaccines worldwide.

ORIGINS OF OPERATION WARP SPEED

While the official Rose Garden launch of OWS took place in May 2020, the planning had been underway for several weeks. Paul Mango, a Trump political appointee who served as deputy chief of staff for policy to Secretary Azar, traces the inception of the effort to March 27, 2020. According to Mango, on that day he and Secretary Azar reviewed the recently executed federal contract with drugmaker Johnson & Johnson to develop a COVID vaccine. The contract amount was nearly a half billion dollars. The lack of urgency built into that contract left both him and Secretary Azar "completely unfulfilled,"[9] Mango later told reporter Dan Diamond in an interview published by POLITICO.

Mango later credited Secretary Azar with being the "architect" of the operation at a vaccine summit conducted at the White House on December 8, 2020, just days before the first shots were to be given.[10] It was Mango, however, who became a central OWS figure and was described by Secretary Azar as the "principal representative" on the effort.[11] Billing himself as the "the foremost leader of Operation Warp Speed," Mango would later write a book about his experience entitled *Warp Speed: Inside the Operation That Beat COVID, the Critics, and the Odds* that was released in March 2021.[12]

Mango's background in both the military and health care consulting made him well suited to coordinate the massive COVID vaccine manufacturing enterprise that would involve both HHS and the DoD. His background in politics also may have prepared him for the highly politicized environment surrounding the entire federal response to the pandemic. In 2017, Mango ran unsuccessfully for the Republican nomination to be governor of Pennsylvania.[13] According to public reporting, he had previously donated over $220,000 to Republican causes and spent over $7 million of his own money in the unsuccessful pursuit of the gubernatorial nomination.[13] Before that run, he had worked for over 20 years as a senior partner at McKinsey & Company. He is a West Point graduate, holds an MBA from Harvard, and served five years in the US Army's 82nd Airborne Division.

Mango described his role in the OWS campaign as being the bridge and liaison between HHS, the DoD, and the White House (author oral interview with Paul Mango, MBA, December 13, 2020). At the White House summit, Mango recounted how he and Azar asked in March 2020 when clinical trials for the COVID vaccine candidates would begin and how they found the FDA's answer, September, to be "completely unsatisfactory."[10] At that point, Mango recounted, Secretary Azar called up some contacts in the pharmaceutical industry and asked, "Who is best vaccine developer in the world?"[10] The name they were given was Dr. Moncef Slaoui, a former executive at GlaxoSmithKline and at that time a member of the Moderna board of directors. After an interview process that included President Trump's son-in-law Jared Kushner, Slaoui was named chief scientist for Operation Warp Speed.

The next day, Secretary Azar called Secretary of Defense Mark Esper and said, "I need a logistics expert," Mango recounted at the White House summit.[10] "That's how we got General Perna." General Gustave Perna is a highly decorated four-star general who at that time oversaw the US Army Materiel Command, the command that manages the global supply chain, synchronizing logistics and sustainment activities across the army.[14] He would be named chief operating officer for Operation Warp Speed.

In another version of the origins of the operation, Dr. Peter Marks, head of the Center for Biologics Evaluation and Research at the FDA, recalls being on a train to a conference in New York City in February 2020. Dr. Marks saw data showing COVID infections had already been recorded on five continents, he later told *USA Today*, and realized that containment would no longer be a viable strategy: "When you can't contain, you mitigate," he said, noting that speed in getting a vaccine developed would be critical.[15]

Dr. Marks and Dr. Robert Kadlec, the HHS assistant secretary for preparedness and response, then wrote a proposal to Secretary Azar in early April.[16] It detailed a process that went from screening potential vaccine candidates to distributing the final product to an estimated 330 million Americans. The plan was based on Marks's experience both working in the pharmaceutical industry and regulating the industry from his position in the FDA.

Their plan contained two of the most critical elements in the eventual success of the vaccine development enterprise. First, it reduced or eliminated financial risk for companies that would be hesitant to engage in expensive research and development at a point when the eventual demand for vaccines was unknown. By providing an infusion of funding, the financial risk to the companies developing vaccines was covered. Second, they created a plan to begin manufacturing of vaccines and simultaneously to conducting clinical trials. In essence, the federal government would foot the bill to manufacture vaccine before knowing whether the product worked. It was a huge gamble, but the bet was that the simultaneous process could make effective vaccines available months earlier than otherwise possible if their safety and effectiveness could be proved.

While Mango credits Secretary Azar with being the architect of OWS, there are others whose streams of thinking went into its inception, reflecting the proverb popularized by President John Kennedy that "victory has one hundred fathers, but defeat is an orphan." Nevertheless, Dr. Janet Woodcock, who was acting director of the FDA and Dr. Marks's boss at that time, gives him primary credit. "The US response to the pandemic as far as vaccines . . . was largely his concept," she told reporter Karen Weintraub.[15] "It was definitely Peter who put the idea together for Operation Warp Speed for vaccines."

Early in the vaccine program's development, as referenced by the president, the project was being internally referred to as Manhattan Project 2, or MP2,[9] in reference to the massive government effort to develop and deploy an atomic weapon during World War II. Mango writes that Marks superseded Azar's MP2 with OWS,[12] a nod to the need for quick work akin to the ability to achieve interstellar travel at light speed as shown in the television and movie series *Star Trek*.

While that name perfectly reflected the urgency needed to stop a global pandemic, it stoked fears by some that in the push for speed, safety would be sacrificed. Its name likely, though inadvertently, contributed to the vaccine hesitancy that significantly stalled progress just a few months after vaccine distribution began. Indeed, a poll conducted by the Associated Press and the NORC Center for Public Affairs Research released shortly after the announcement of OWS in May 2020 showed that only half of Americans would take a vaccine if scientists successfully developed one.[17] Of those polled, 30% said they were unsure, and close to 20% said that they would definitely not take a COVID shot. In contrast, the vaccine uptake for routine childhood immunizations such as measles, chickenpox, and polio annually exceeds 90%.[18] Clear early warning signs on looming vaccine hesitancy thus appear to have been largely overlooked in the warp speed planning at that time. We return to this issue as we examine vaccine hesitancy in more depth in a subsequent chapter.

DEFINING THE MISSION

Vaccine distribution and administration is far more complicated than shipping boxes around the country, even when those shipments must maintain certain ultracold temperatures and be tracked minute by minute in terms of location. Distribution includes repackaging large quantities for shipments to smaller clinical sites, providing instructions on how to administer the vaccine itself, and coordinating ancillary supplies such as syringes to administer the vaccine. Attention to product expiration dates and handling of expired doses are also factors. Distribution during OWS also included planning to expand the pool of eligible vaccinators and advance consideration of how to address potential vaccine hesitancy.

Instead of embracing these considerations, however, it seems as if early on the operation's military planners adopted a narrow definition of their mission to simply deliver vaccines to a specified point, as they would battle supplies. This perspective fundamentally misunderstood the subtleties and nuances of administering a brand-new medical product to the entire country and the massive communications effort that would be needed to educate Americans about how the new vaccine was developed, tested, and approved. Americans would need precise information about when the vaccine would become available, who would be prioritized to receive it first, and how they could find and schedule an appointment at a convenient point of administration.

The military and HHS political appointees forming the operation's leadership team understandably focused on overcoming the massive vaccine development and manufacturing challenges. Yet as they began to plan for distribution, they seemed to overlook many of the assumptions of public health planners at CDC and in the states. These assumptions included the vital need to focus on coordinating early and often to overcome the implementation challenges in getting the vaccine delivered over the proverbial last mile, or from the distribution point into people's arms. Central to this challenge was understanding that trust was essential to creating demand for vaccine. This encompasses trust in its safety, trust in its effectiveness, and trust that the vaccine is even necessary in the first place.

As we describe in a subsequent chapter, shipping vaccines to various locations without a commensurate effort to build trust in the vaccines themselves led to vaccine hesitancy and refusal in many parts of the United States. Public health officials who had studied John Barry's *The Great Influenza* were acutely aware that the biggest lesson from the 1918 global influenza pandemic was that broken trust led to the fraying of society, not lack of mitigation or containment efforts. "In 1918, pressured to maintain wartime morale, neither national nor local government officials told the truth," Barry wrote in a 2020 op-ed in the *New York Times*.[19] In an uncanny parallel to 1918, President Trump, pressured to maintain morale and buoy the economy in the lead-up to his 2020 election campaign for a second term, purposely downplayed the seriousness of COVID and minimized the need for comprehensive public health action. His megaphone was so loud and his attacks on experts and "the doctors" were so effective that they drowned out those who tried to set the record straight.[20,21] The impact of this false information and downplaying of the severity of the virus early in the crisis continues to be felt long after.

MORE THAN A MATH PROBLEM

Days after General Perna's appointment on May 15, 2020, the *New York Times* published an article with some of his first public comments on the challenges he envisioned being part of Operation Warp Speed.[22] The general noted that President Trump said that the goal of the project was to distribute a vaccine "prior to the end of the year."[22] He also affirmed that Trump was relying on the DoD to manage the manufacturing logistics related to vaccine development. In the interview, the general said discussions about the equipment and facilities needed for production were just beginning. The *Times* reported:

> Gen. Gustave F. Perna . . . described his work as a "math problem": how to get 300 million doses of a vaccine that doesn't yet exist to Americans—by January. Finding the supplies and planning their distribution would occur at the same time, [Perna] said. "I need to have syringes," General Perna said. "I need to have wipes, right? I need to have Band-Aids. I need to have the vaccine." He added: "Now, how am I going to distribute it? What is it going to be distributed in? What do I need to order now to make sure I have the distribution capability? The small bottles, the trucks."[23]

Notably absent in General Perna's first interview on his new mission was any indication that he had been briefed on the federal government's existing plans and capacity to distribute vaccine during pandemics. His remarks were an early indication that the government saw the challenge in terms of manufacturing and logistics, not the administration of the vaccine in people's arms. There was no mention of building upon how the CDC annually coordinates distribution of millions of doses of routine childhood vaccines and also supports private-sector distribution of tens of millions of annual doses of flu vaccine.[23] Reflecting a Trump administration aversion to utilizing anything from prior administrations, there was no reference to building on vaccine plans provided in the Obama-era *Playbook for Early Response to High-Consequence Emerging Infectious Disease Threats and Biological Incidents*,[24,25] nor was there any mention of the HHS *National Strategy for Pandemic Influenza*,[26] issued under President Bush first in 2005 and last updated in 2017.[27]

To many public health professionals, General Perna's public comments made it appear that he thought he would need to start from scratch. Moreover, referring to the challenge simply as a math problem struck many as his failure to understand the nuance of behavioral science in creating demand and introducing a brand-new vaccine. To be sure, General Perna had strong supporters. "Perna is the best logistician in the US government," Dr. Nelson Michael, director of the Center for Infectious Disease Research at the Walter Reed Army Institute of Research told CNN.[28] "You have the entire weight of a four-star general who knows how to move bullets and beans from Point A to Point B and get them there at the right time."

The concerns about his appointment, according to some public health experts, was that there is a big difference between delivering battle supplies and shots of a vaccine. Most battle supplies are not based on a brand-new medical technology; they don't need to be injected; they don't require ultracold storage handling; they don't require recipients to return three weeks later for a second dose; their consumption doesn't have to be recorded in one of the 59 different state and territorial information systems; and there is not an active, organized movement opposing their consumption and spreading misinformation about them. In addition, the diverse nature of state and local public health systems and the multiple stakeholders that administer vaccines at the local level makes centralized, top-down planning that may work in military environments very difficult in the decentralized public health and health care sectors.

Following the OWS announcement and after subsequent media interviews with General Perna, some in the public health community worried that the president had placed an individual in charge of vaccine distribution who had little apparent knowledge about the existing vaccine system and capacities of state health agencies and their health care partners. Nor did it seem he had familiarity with the federal, state, and local public health agencies that have over 60 years of experience running immunization programs. In fairness to the general, he could not have expected to be familiar with these systems, as they were not within his purview as head of the US Army Materiel Command. His logistics skill set was focused on getting military supplies to troops at bases around the world. The question was, Would this translate to delivering a medical product, not to far-flung military bases, but to every community across the nation?

John Auerbach, the former state health officer for Massachusetts and then-CEO at the Trust for America's Health later summed up the concern: "Military personnel won't be familiar with the health resources available in a community. They don't know who the doctors are or where the community health centers are located or what resources they have. They don't know where the pharmacies are. Public health people do know, that's part of what they do."[29] Furthermore, public health professionals experienced in vaccine distribution knew that the challenges of vaccine distribution go beyond logistics. There is a complex interplay of behavioral science and risk communication that come into play as well that involves knowing what messages build trust and what messages exacerbate vaccine hesitancy.

Public health officials know that who delivers the message can be just as important as the content itself, and they know the existing capacity at local levels to deliver both messages and health services. None of these considerations were reflected in the early public messaging around Operation Warp Speed, and there was no specific mention of the role the CDC would play. To better understand the operation's strategy and the anticipated role of state and local health agencies, the leaders of national public health associations representing health officials and immunization leaders (i.e., Association of State and Territorial Health Officials, National Association of County and City Health Officials, Association of Immunization Managers, and American Immunization Registry Association) reached out to the operation's newly announced leaders a few weeks after they were announced.

In a letter sent on June 23, 2020, the associations praised the government administration's commitment to developing a vaccine and wrote, "We want to offer our support, expertise, experience, and partnership, which we believe will be crucial to planning and executing a successful national COVID-19 vaccine program."[30]

Because the announcement of the OWS operation made no mention of the nation's existing immunization infrastructure and systems to distribute vaccine, the public health groups offered recommendations to build upon existing plans and to avoid duplication. The associations also noted the importance of clarifying the expected role of the military. Citing survey data that more than one-quarter of Americans polled said they would definitely not get a COVID vaccine if it were available, they asked to work together on building vaccine confidence.

The letter closed with a strong recommendation on the importance of managing expectations and shared a key lesson from the experience with the 2009 H1N1 influenza vaccine distribution. Citing a Government Accounting Office report written on lessons learned from the 2009 response, they wrote, "The credibility of all levels of government was diminished when the amount of vaccine available to the public in October 2009 did not meet expectations set by federal officials."[31(p2)] It was a lesson doomed to be ignored.

The associations' letter closed by seeking to further enhance the close coordination and cooperation between federal, state, local, and tribal authorities that would be necessary to achieve the operation's success. It noted that experts in public health agency leadership and immunization program management shared their goals and stood ready to bring their experience and commitment to the campaign. The letter was addressed to both Dr. Slaoui and General Perna as the operation's coleads. It included copies to Vice President Mike Pence, Dr. Deborah Birx, HHS secretary Alex Azar, CDC director Dr. Robert Redfield, CDC's National Center for Immunization and Respiratory Diseases director Dr. Nancy Messonnier, and the National Institutes of Health's Dr. Anthony Fauci.

In a continuation of the Trump administration leaders' failure to communicate directly with the state and local officials on the front lines of the pandemic, it never received a response.

Regarding the lack of response to the national associations' outreach, Claire Hannan, executive director of the Association of Immunization Managers, recalled, "We were baffled. Why wouldn't they want to talk to the experts? It only became clear in retrospect that they had an ideological preference for the private sector over the public sector. And by extension, the loss of trust in CDC meant that there was a loss of trust in us" (author interview with Claire Hannan, MPH, December 28, 2021).

Meanwhile, Operation Warp Speed planning continued to push forward with limited engagement of those expected to administer the vaccine, focusing on speed and logistics, paying little heed to the current system of vaccine distribution. This focus would create problems for the team in the later rollout of vaccines, where implementation and operational realities took over. These included communications challenges concerning vaccine production and allocation, failure to account for the barriers that vaccine clinics and pharmacies would encounter as they administered vaccines, and an urgent challenge to build confidence in the new vaccines. It seemed as if previous planning assumptions about the role of public health agencies in pandemic response were being changed, or warped, and public health officials became increasingly worried.

REFERENCES

1. National Archives and Records Administration. Remarks by President Trump on vaccine development. May 15, 2020. Available at: https://trumpwhitehouse.archives.gov/briefings-statements/remarks-president-trump-vaccine-development. Accessed September 11, 2022.

2. Herper M, Florko N. Drug makers rebut Trump tweet that FDA "deep state" is delaying Covid-19 vaccines and drugs. *STAT*. August 22, 2020. Available at: https://www.statnews.com/2020/08/22/drug-makers-rebut-trump-tweet-that-fda-deep-state-delaying-covid19-vaccines-drugs. Accessed September 11, 2022.

3. Soucheray S. Fauci: vaccine at least year away, as COVID-19 death toll rises to 9 in Seattle. *CIDRAP*. March 3, 2020. Available at: https://www.cidrap.umn.edu/news-perspective/2020/03/fauci-vaccine-least-year-away-covid-19-death-toll-rises-9-seattle. Accessed September 11, 2022.

4. Sun LH, Dawsey J. CDC feels pressure from Trump as rift grows over coronavirus response. *Washington Post*. July 9, 2020. Available at: https://www.washingtonpost.com/health/trump-sidelines-public-health-advisers-in-growing-rift-over-coronavirus-response/2020/07/09/ad803218-c12a-11ea-9fdd-b7ac6b051dc8_story.html. Accessed September 11, 2022.

5. Centers for Disease Control and Prevention, National Center for Immunization and Respiratory Diseases. Pandemic vaccine program: distribution, tracking, administration, and monitoring. 2020. Available at: https://www.cdc.gov/flu/pdf/pandemic-resources/pandemic-influenza-vaccine-distribution-9p-508.pdf. Accessed September 11, 2022.

6. Centers for Disease Control and Prevention. Final estimates for 2009–10 seasonal influenza and influenza A (H1N1) 2009 monovalent vaccination coverage—United States, August 2009 through May, 2010. May 13, 2011. Available at: https://www.cdc.gov/flu/fluvaxview/coverage_0910estimates.htm. Accessed September 11, 2022.

7. Kollewe J. Pfizer accused of pandemic profiteering as profits double. *Guardian*. February 8, 2022. Available at: https://www.theguardian.com/business/2022/feb/08/pfizer-covid-vaccine-pill-profits-sales. Accessed September 11, 2022.

8. Grossman M, Loftus P. Moderna beats profit estimates, fueled by Covid-19 vaccine sales. *Wall Street Journal*. February 24, 2022. Available at: https://www.wsj.com/articles/moderna-beats-profit-estimates-fueled-by-vaccine-sales-11645707646. Accessed September 11, 2022.

9. Diamond D. The crash landing of "Operation Warp Speed." *Politico*. January 17, 2021. Available at: https://www.politico.com/news/2021/01/17/crash-landing-of-operation-warp-speed-459892. Accessed September 11, 2022.

10. US Department of State. White House Operation Warp Speed vaccine summit. December 8, 2020. Available at: https://www.youtube.com/watch?v=0yclESPhfIU. Accessed September 11, 2022.

11. Olson L. Former PA. guv candidate Paul Mango at the center of Trump admin's vaccine push. *Pennsylvania Capital-Star*. October 26, 2020. https://www.penncapital-star.com/covid-19/former-pa-guv-candidate-paul-mango-at-the-center-of-trump-admins-vaccine-push. Accessed September 11, 2022.

12. Mango P. *Warp Speed: Inside the Operation That Beat COVID, the Critics, and the Odds.* New York, NY: Republic Book Publishers; 2022.

13. Potter C. Who is Paul Mango and why, in his words, can he beat Tom Wolf for governor? *Pittsburgh Post-Gazette.* May 17, 2017. Available at: https://www.post-gazette.com/early-returns/erstate/2017/05/17/Who-is-Paul-Mango/stories/201705170188. Accessed September 11, 2022.

14. Army Materiel Command. AMC—the army's materiel integrator. Available at: https://www.amc.army.mil. Accessed September 11, 2022.

15. Weintraub K. Behind the historic US vaccine effort is FDA's Peter Marks. The job is "not for the faint of heart." *USA Today.* June 23, 2021. Available at: https://www.usatoday.com/story/news/health/2021/06/23/fda-peter-marks-behind-us-covid-vaccination-effort/7681024002. Accessed September 11, 2022.

16. Abutaleb Y, McGinley L, Johnson CY. How the "deep state" scientists vilified by Trump helped him deliver an unprecedented achievement. *Washington Post.* December 14, 2020. Available at: https://www.washingtonpost.com/health/2020/12/14/trump-operation-warp-speed-vaccine. Accessed September 11, 2022.

17. Neergaard L, Fingerhut H. AP-NORC poll: half of Americans would get a COVID-19 vaccine. *AP News.* May 27, 2020. Available at: https://apnews.com/article/donald-trump-us-news-ap-top-news-politics-virus-outbreak-dacdc8bc428dd4df6511bfa259cfec44. Accessed September 11, 2022.

18. Centers for Disease Control and Prevention. FastStats: immunization. August 3, 2021. Available at: https://www.cdc.gov/nchs/fastats/immunize.htm. Accessed September 11, 2022.

19. Barry JM. The single most important lesson from the 1918 influenza. *New York Times.* March 17, 2020. Available at: https://www.nytimes.com/2020/03/17/opinion/coronavirus-1918-spanish-flu.html. Accessed September 11, 2022.

20. Cathey L. With string of attacks on doctors and experts, Trump takes aim at science: analysis. *ABC News.* August 6, 2020. Available at: https://abcnews.go.com/Politics/string-attacks-doctors-experts-trump-takes-aim-science/story?id=72170408. Accessed September 11, 2022.

21. Birx DL. *Silent Invasion: The Untold Story of the Trump Administration, Covid-19, and Preventing the Next Pandemic Before It's Too Late.* New York, NY: Harper, an imprint of HarperCollins Publishers; 2022.

22. Zimmer C, Sheikh K, Weiland N. A new entry in the race for a coronavirus vaccine: hope. *New York Times.* May 20, 2020. Available at: https://www.nytimes.com/2020/05/20/health/coronavirus-vaccines.html. Accessed September 11, 2022.

23. Centers for Disease Control and Prevention. Seasonal influenza vaccine supply & distribution. March 7, 2022. Available at: https://www.cdc.gov/flu/prevent/vaccine-supply-distribution.htm. Accessed September 11, 2022.

24. Executive Office of the President of the United States. Playbook for early response to high-consequence emerging infectious disease threats and biological incidents. 2016. Available at: https://www.documentcloud.org/documents/6819268-Pandemic-Playbook. Accessed September 11, 2022.

25. Knight V. Evidence shows Obama team left a pandemic "game plan" for Trump administration. *Kaiser Health News.* May 15, 2020. Available at: https://khn.org/news/evidence-shows-obama-team-left-a-pandemic-game-plan-for-trump-administration. Accessed September 11, 2022.

26. Homeland Security Council. National strategy for pandemic influenza. November 2005. Available at: https://www.cdc.gov/flu/pandemic-resources/pdf/pandemic-influenza-strategy-2005.pdf. Accessed September 11, 2022.

27. US Department of Health and Human Services. Pandemic influenza plan, 2017 update. 2017. Available at: https://www.cdc.gov/flu/pandemic-resources/pdf/pan-flu-report-2017v2.pdf. Accessed September 11, 2022.

28. Cohen E, Bonifield J, Jenkins S. Pfizer's ultra-cold vaccine, a "very complex" distribution plan and an exploding head emoji. *CNN*. November 10, 2020. Available at: https://www.cnn.com/2020/11/10/health/pfizer-vaccine-distribution-cold-chain/index.html. Accessed September 11, 2022.

29. Florko N. New document reveals scope and structure of Operation Warp Speed and underscores vast military involvement. *STAT*. September 28, 2020. Available at: https://www.statnews.com/2020/09/28/operation-warp-speed-vast-military-involvement. Accessed September 11, 2022.

30. Association of State and Territorial Health Offices, American Immunization Registry Association, National Association of County and City Health Officials, Association of Immunization Managers. Letter to General Perna and Dr. Slaoui. June 23, 2020. Available at: https://www.naccho.org/uploads/downloadable-resources/Letter-to-Operation-Warp-Speed-Leaders.pdf. Accessed September 11, 2022.

31. US Government Accountability Office. Influenza pandemic: lessons from the H1N1 pandemic should be incorporated into future planning. June 27, 2011. Available at: https://www.gao.gov/products/gao-11-632. Accessed September 11, 2022.

4

Warp Speed Warps Planning

Every American who wants the vaccine will be able to get the vaccine. And we think by spring we're going to be in a position that nobody would have believed possible just a few months ago. (Applause.) Yeah. Amazing. Really amazing. They say it's—they say it's somewhat of a miracle, and I think that's true . . . Later today, General Gus Perna will outline the detailed plan to rapidly distribute the vaccine to every state, territory, and tribe. States have designated over 50,000 sites that will receive the vaccine. We've worked very closely with the states.[1]

–President Donald Trump, Operation Warp Speed Vaccine Summit,
December 8, 2020

Very clearly by January 20, this will be a mop-up operation. All the heavy lifting will have been done. The flow of vaccines will have been out there for four to six weeks.[2]

–Paul Mango, December 3, 2020

On April 23, 2020, just four months into the global pandemic and a month before the formal launch of Operation Warp Speed (OWS), the Centers for Disease Control and Prevention (CDC) issued a three-page memorandum to state and local immunization programs. The memo offered the first official communication from the federal government to inform COVID vaccine distribution planning. It offered a glimmer of hope that the path out of the pandemic was about to be paved.

A cover note from Dr. Melinda Wharton, director of the Immunization Services Branch of the CDC's Center for Immunization and Respiratory Diseases, said, "Fortunately, public health has been thinking through and preparing for pandemic vaccination efforts for many years, and now is the time to review, update and modify pandemic vaccination plans."[3] In other words, the nation did not need to start from scratch.

However, in many regards, the national planning did just that. In the wake of President Trump's launch of OWS, three men were placed in direct charge of vaccine distribution who had no formal training in medicine or public health, had no experience with the public health system or prior pandemic response, and up to that point had not made any public announcements about vaccine distribution planning. The three were Paul Mango, General Gus Perna, and Lieutenant General Paul Ostrowski. Paul Mango was a corporate consultant and political appointee who later billed himself as the "the foremost leader of Operation Warp Speed."[4] He was also Department of Health and Human Services (HHS) secretary Alex Azar's key representative to the planning group. General Perna, a four-star general who previously served as the 19th commanding general of US Army Materiel

Command, was named chief operating officer. And, under General Perna, Lieutenant General Ostrowski was appointed to be OWS director of supply, production, and distribution. Like Mango, Ostrowski is a West Point graduate who served 35 years in the US Army. His final assignment on active army duty was as the principal military deputy and director of the Army Acquisition Corps, where he oversaw a $36 billion portfolio of defense material acquisitions.

There is no doubt that these talented OWS leaders had great skills, but in their new roles they had a lot to learn about the complexities of vaccine development and distribution. In retrospect, it was inevitable that there would be a culture clash between the military's culture of command and control and public health's significantly different culture of collaboration and community engagement. The physical distance separating OWS leaders and experts at the CDC was symbolic of this rift. Whereas OWS was based in Washington, DC, close to the action and in the thick of the day-to-day pressures facing key leaders in the national COVID response, CDC experts were based 600 miles away in Atlanta, Georgia.

Indeed, from the outset, OWS officials exerted authority over career public health professionals who had decades of experience managing immunization programs and overseeing the distribution and administration of vaccines. The military push was to get as much vaccine out as quickly as possible to "defeat the enemy,"[5] to win the COVID war. Public health leaders shared that desire to win, but when they pushed for planning to incorporate experience from earlier pandemic vaccine responses, they were perceived by OWS as contributing to the slow grind of bureaucratic decision-making.

Drawing on lessons from H1N1 and the experience of managing the nation's routine vaccine distribution process, public health leaders wanted to make sure that the rollout was credible, that the first weeks of the rollout allowed state health departments to recalibrate and course correct as needed, that the public's expectations as to when they could be vaccinated would be set realistically, and that state and local public health collaborators had what they needed to succeed. But public health's goals were seen as roadblocks to the rapid distribution of an urgently needed vaccine, a vaccine that many Trump administration officials had promised would be available to tens of millions of Americans as soon it was developed.

To stem the impact of the culture clash, the CDC's Dr. Nancy Messonnier reportedly sent an email to OWS leaders on May 27, 2020, looking to bridge this cultural divide, writing, "Part of the struggle here is rapidly mashing together two cultures. I am hoping that a joint work plan will go a long way to setting up swim lanes, timelines, and deliverables."[6] Unfortunately, her attempt to bridge the cultures was unsuccessful.

There is a great deal that the OWS campaign got right, and for that these leaders and their teams deserve immense credit. The experience, capacity, and skill they brought to mobilize vaccine manufacturing, requisition necessary supplies, and swiftly execute myriad contracts with necessary partners was impressive and most likely would have been incredibly difficult to do for anyone without the logistics and procurement credentials of the Department of Defense (DoD) as part of the OWS team. One CDC official we spoke to told us that the US Army "kicked down every barrier there was so the US government could purchase everything necessary to vaccinate every American" (author interview with senior CDC official, March 28, 2022). Many public health leaders recognized that the task of vaccine distribution was so large and complex that it could not have been accomplished without the mobilization and support of the military. A senior public health official we interviewed even asserted that the vaccine distribution effort could not have succeeded without General Perna at the helm.

In our interview with him, Mr. James Blumenstock, who most recently served as senior vice president for pandemic response and recovery at the Association of State and Territorial Health Officials and is one of the nation's top experts on public health agency preparedness and response programs, recalled that at first he was not too concerned about the military's involvement in OWS. He thought that military involvement made a lot of sense and had observed that many state public health preparedness programs had hired military veterans to help run state emergency operations centers (author interview with James Blumenstock, MA, December 2, 2021). Their attention to detail, understanding of how to implement a chain of command, and experience under fire were all attributes that enhanced public health preparedness. But by placing political appointees and military leaders without public health or vaccine experience in authority over the experienced professionals of the CDC, President Trump introduced unnecessary conflict and confusion. While wildly successful in speeding the development and manufacture of safe, effective vaccines in record time, the creation of OWS may, ironically, have slowed critical CDC vaccine distribution planning for months.

On the basis of our observations and interviews with federal, state, and local officials, we identified five critical challenges that impeded the vaccine distribution planning process. These challenges then became largely responsible for the problems in the initial rollout. Some of them had deleterious effects on the campaign long after the original OWS leadership had moved on. We review these challenges, not to point fingers or assess blame, but to document improvements to response that could be applied when a future pandemic calls for another nationwide vaccination campaign. Without question, OWS is a great American achievement with global consequences, especially in the areas of vaccine development and manufacturing. Our critique should not take away from that achievement. We especially underscore our belief that all the leaders and colleagues referenced herein were working to the best of their ability, with incomplete information, under incredibly difficult circumstances, and with total dedication to serving the country.

In our review, these were the five challenges that impeded the vaccine distribution planning process:

1. Public health inexperience and the hubris of top OWS leaders that discounted and temporarily sidelined the CDC lead to major delays as state and local partners waited for shared planning assumptions and federal guidance.

2. Top OWS leaders defined the mission and its operations too narrowly.
3. Officials delayed the engagement of public health leaders in state and local jurisdictions.
4. Top OWS officials allocated federal funds generously to private corporations to get the vaccines developed but not to the public agencies critical to ensuring success in the critical last mile where vaccine administration takes place.
5. Lack of respect for career public health officials delayed the planning process, although in the end OWS essentially adapted the distribution plan established by the CDC and states.

Each of these features is explored in more detail below.

INEXPERIENCE AND HUBRIS SIDELINED THE CENTERS FOR DISEASE CONTROL AND PREVENTION

None of the three top leaders overseeing vaccine distribution (Perna, Ostrowski, and Mango) had any training in medicine, public health, or vaccines, so it would be natural to think that they would quickly turn to career civil servants at the CDC with that experience. However, from the outset, the CDC's leading vaccine experts along with state and local immunization program managers would report being largely excluded from the overall OWS planning process. When consulted, CDC contributors reported that their professional judgments and recommendations were ignored, second-guessed, or dismissed as being too deliberative or too time consuming (author interview with senior CDC official, March 28, 2022).[2,6]

Despite being conceived of and billed as a partnership between the DoD and the HHS, it was perhaps ironic that the HHS operating division with the most experience in vaccine distribution, CDC, was initially excluded from the vaccine distribution planning and decision-making. Largely as a result of their assessment of CDC's early missteps in handling the COVID testing enterprise, senior appointed leaders at HHS headquarters as well as in the White House developed a distrust of CDC and aversion to engaging the experienced professionals they needed most to succeed.

The marginalization of CDC began early. While himself a civilian, Paul Mango, the deputy chief of staff at HHS charged with coordinating the effort with DoD, was a West Point graduate and former army ranger. That background may explain a lot about his bias to promote the views of the US Army over public health. In an interview for this book, Mango was open about why the CDC did not initially have a central role: "Part of the issue was they [CDC] were 600 miles away in Atlanta. If you are going to have a single team and break down barriers, sometimes getting people together is a really good thing," he said (author interview with Paul Mango, MBA, December 13, 2021). "We had a reception for all the HHS folks to meet the DoD folks—and people would also ask me 'Paul, why have all these guys in camo fatigues descended on the building?'" He continued:

We got them together to meet each other and it worked—but the CDC was down in Atlanta, and it was hard for them to participate in that. I think part of it was [also] that in the early days of the pandemic the CDC was viewed as having failed at several things; laboratory testing was the big one. So there had been some lost confidence there. (Author interview with Paul Mango, MBA, December 13, 2021.)

An organizational chart[7] that emerged later showed that Lieutenant General Ostrowski reported to General Perna, who in turn reported to Secretaries Azar (HHS) and Esper (Defense). Except for Secretary Azar, who is a lawyer and former pharmaceutical executive, none had ever even worked with the state and local public health agencies that would be on the front lines coordinating vaccine distribution. Adding confusion over who was in charge of vaccine distribution and administration, President Trump had named Dr. Moncef Slaoui as the OWS campaign's chief scientific advisor. Given that Dr. Slaoui was an expert in vaccine development, it was unclear what his role would be in advising on vaccine distribution or working with the public health sector.

To be fair, the military leaders put in charge of the operation did not seek this mission. The essential problem was the belief that extensive logistical experience supporting combat operations in the Middle East over the past 20 years could be straightforwardly applied to domestic vaccine distribution. On top of this, civilian and US Army OWS leaders brought to the planning table an ideologically driven, preconceived, and explicit preference for the private sector over the public sector. In summary, OWS was going to rely on the speed, efficiency, and innovation of private industry and not on the scientific advice of career technocrats, who were viewed as slowing down the campaign's marching cadence.

Some top leaders' views on CDC experts were crystalized in a statement made by Michael Caputo, the HHS assistant secretary for public affairs, who shared on Facebook his belief that CDC staff "haven't gotten out of their sweatpants except for meetings at coffee shops," at which they plan "how they're going to attack Donald Trump next . . . There are scientists who work for this government who do not want America to get well, not until after Joe Biden is president."[8]

From the perspective of state and local public health officials, one of the central issues to resolve early in OWS work was whether the federal government would utilize the existing vaccine distribution system or would pursue a new distribution structure. States could not move forward with any substantive planning without this critical information. President Trump's Rose Garden announcement that the military would oversee vaccine distribution cast significant doubt on whether existing pandemic vaccination plans utilizing the existing system and led by the CDC would be followed. For at least three months following this announcement, state and local health officials were largely left in the dark about this and other critical issues regarding their distribution and administration plans.

Claire Hannan has three decades of experience in support of state and local immunization programs and is one of the nation's most experienced leaders in vaccine distribution and the programs that make it work. Recalling this period she said, "There was just a lot of confusion. And during that time frame, nothing could get accomplished. The states could not develop a process to enroll providers, they could not educate providers, and they could not build out their tracking systems. They didn't know what data elements would be required. They just weren't able to do all of the things that you would want to be done ahead of time . . . And also they didn't have any money" (author interview with Claire Hannan, MPH, March 17, 2022).

General Perna demonstrated his lack of understanding of the existing American vaccine delivery enterprise in a candid admission on the national news program *60 Minutes* broadcast on November 9, 2020, close to six months after he was appointed to lead OWS and a month before the first COVID vaccines were delivered. In his interview, he first alleged that no vaccine planning had occurred before his appointment despite at least a decade of pandemic influenza vaccine planning done at HHS and CDC, stating, "There was no doctrine, there was no strategy, there was no structure of people to this end."[9] This likely came as a surprise and insult to the 720 public health professionals who work in CDC's National Center for Immunization and Respiratory Diseases (NCIRD) who are committed to the mission of the prevention of disease, disability, and death through immunization and by control of respiratory and related diseases, as well as thousands of public health workers in the states who oversee the vaccination of Americans every day.

What General Perna said next was perhaps even more shocking. Pointing to a sheet of pharmaceutical-related acronyms taped to the wall in Perna's office, *60 Minutes* reporter David Martin said, "You have a cheat sheet here. This is all the drug jargon."[9] General Perna replied, "It is. I listen every day to what is being said, and then I spend a good part of my evening Googling these words, so that I can participate preferably at an intellectual level, but at least at an understanding." It was a stunning admission that the man placed in charge by Donald Trump of the most important vaccination campaign in a century was still learning the basics of vaccine jargon. General Perna is an honorable and intelligent man with a lifetime of service to the nation. But the question must be asked, How much faster could the OWS vaccine distribution planning have occurred if the leader was not spending evenings learning the basics of the product he oversaw distributing?

It might be reasonable to think that given this lack of experience in vaccine distribution, OWS leaders would seek out and defer to the expertise in CDC. It is, after all, the agency that oversees the distribution of vaccines every year from every vaccine manufacturer to health departments and private health providers across the country and has done so since 1962. Instead, the CDC officials with the nation's most experience in vaccine distribution were initially undermined in their efforts to develop a workable partnership and plan. It started with the formulation of the OWS board of directors. Mango described how the directors designed a governance structure to "bypass the slow grind of bureaucratic decision-making."[4(p15)] This included only the "essential players"[4(p15)]—those from HHS, the DoD, and the White House. The OWS board of directors apparently did include Dr. Robert Redfield, though by this point in the pandemic it was apparent that he was not at all effective in conveying or advocating for the prerogatives of his agency's immunization experts. And while he was a respected virologist, Dr. Redfield's background largely focused on laboratory research rather than public health practice, with little direct experience in vaccine distribution.

One of the top government officials with that experience was Dr. Nancy Messonnier. At the time, she led a center within CDC with hundreds of staff experienced in distributing tens of millions of vaccines to both children and adults. As noted, prior to the formation of OWS, she and her team had already begun adapting CDC's pandemic vaccination plans and had issued an initial planning assumptions memo to the states on April 23, 2020.[3]

Dr. Messonnier is a leading global expert on vaccines and respiratory diseases. She was one of the people best prepared to lead and guide COVID vaccine distribution. She received her BA from the University of Pennsylvania and after receiving her MD from the University of Chicago School of Medicine completed her internal medicine residency training at the University of Pennsylvania. She began her public health career in 1995 as a CDC Epidemic Intelligence Service officer and subsequently held several leadership posts across the CDC. Before being appointed director of the NCIRD, she served as acting director for the Center for Preparedness and Response, deputy director of the NCIRD, acting director of the Division of Global Health Protection in the Center for Global Health, and chief of the Meningitis and Vaccine Preventable Diseases Branch in NCIRD.

On the global stage, Dr. Messonnier played a pivotal role in the successful public-private partnership to develop and implement a low-cost vaccine to prevent epidemic meningococcal meningitis in Africa—more than 150 million people in the African meningitis belt have been vaccinated with MenAfriVac since 2010. With remarkable impact, Dr. Messonnier also has been a leader in CDC's preparedness and response to anthrax, including during the 2001 intentional anthrax release and in evaluating simplified schedules for use of a licensed anthrax vaccine. She spearheaded CDC's Vaccinate with Confidence initiative, which includes activities aimed at reaching communities with low flu vaccination rates or high likelihood of COVID complications such as African American and Hispanic communities. She has written more than 140 articles and chapters and has received numerous awards.[10] As head of the NCIRD, she had direct oversight of the immunization programs across the country.

By many accounts, Dr. Messonnier and her CDC team were the most qualified people in the US government to design and oversee COVID vaccine distribution. Early in the pandemic, however, she made the unfortunate mistake of telling the truth about COVID in an administration seeking to downplay it. During CDC telebriefings on COVID, Dr. Messonnier was one of the only officials to warn the public that the United States should prepare for an unprecedented health crisis: "Ultimately, we expect we will see community spread in this country. It's not so much a question of if this will happen anymore but rather more a question of exactly when this will happen and how many people in this country will have severe illness."[11]

The frankness of her remarks, including her February 25, 2020, warning that COVID could cause "severe" disruptions to everyday life,[12] angered the president while he was on an overseas trip to India and provoked the ire of other officials in the White House who were downplaying the seriousness of the threat. Dr. Messonnier's prescient warnings triggered a plunge in the stock market, with an immediate 3.4% drop in the Dow Jones Industrial Average. According to reporting by the *Washington Post*, the incident so enraged President Trump that he directed aides to counter her warning and repeatedly asked for her to be fired.[13] Thereafter, she was largely removed from visible roles in the agency's briefings despite her astute prediction and years of experience with vaccine-preventable diseases.

Despite being sidelined, however, Dr. Messonnier and her staff persisted. She remained at her post, rallied her team, and tried to set a tone within CDC that business as usual would not be adequate to prepare for the nation's most massive vaccine distribution programs (author interview with senior CDC official, March 28, 2022). As soon as the OWS team was in place, she and her staff began to educate their new military colleagues on the nuances and challenges that needed to be fully considered in the OWS distribution plans. By many accounts, things got off to a rocky start.

One of the earliest challenges was that neither she nor her boss, CDC director Dr. Robert Redfield, was invited to the daily OWS board of directors meetings convened by Paul Mango. An OWS organizational chart showed that either by design or oversight, Dr. Messonnier was buried in the chain of command, with her reporting to Ostrowski, who reported to Perna.[7] Even so, she was the only CDC official and one of the very few women to appear anywhere on the organizational chart of the greatest and most challenging vaccination campaign in history.

Instead, the chart revealed that four generals and roughly 56 additional military officials were involved in the leadership of the OWS campaign. Reporter Nicholas Florko's analysis in *STAT* showed only a third (29) of the roughly 90 leaders on the chart were not employed by the DoD, with most of them being detailed from other operational divisions within HHS.[7] A subsequent review by the Government Accountability Office (GAO) found that as of September 2021, DoD had assigned 76 officials from the Army, Navy, Air Force, and Marine Corps to work on OWS.[14(p7)] Officials at HHS told GAO that their department generally did not assign a specific number of staff to work directly on the effort but stated that hundreds of officials from various HHS agencies, such as the Office of the Assistant Secretary for Preparedness and Response, CDC, and National Institutes of Health, have worked on OWS-related efforts. That was indeed true, but very few had leadership roles in the project and visibility on policy setting and day-to-day decision-making.

Why did the relationship between OWS and CDC get off to a rocky start? Paul Mango offers a compelling insider's view of how they put together an extraordinary team and achieved what many experts thought was impossible: developing, manufacturing, and distributing a safe and effective vaccine in record time. In his book, published in March 2022 after he left the federal government, Mango describes how early in the planning process "tension emerged" between the US Army and the CDC, with the CDC having "a strong preference for using the nation's public health agencies to both distribute *and administer* the vaccine [emphasis added]."[4] US Army leaders preferred using the private sector.

But contrary to Mango's account, so did CDC and state public health partners: for decades the CDC and their state partners have distributed publicly financed vaccines largely through private-sector health care providers. In 2008, the CDC contracted with a private pharmaceutical distribution company called McKesson to be the central distributor of vaccines through the federal Vaccines for Children (VFC) program. This company served as a centralized vaccine distributor during the H1N1 flu pandemic in 2009.[15] Later, the CDC added an addendum to the contract with McKesson to scale up for vaccine distribution in any future pandemic. During the H1N1 influenza outbreak in 2009, the CDC and its state public health partners also pioneered the distribution of flu vaccines via pharmacies. In other words, the CDC had always envisioned private-sector support to distribute vaccines to most of the population, with governmental clinics providing the safety net.

The real source of tension was that in their efforts to bypass the bureaucracy and cut red tape, OWS leaders initially minimized the role of the CDC, which since the beginning of the pandemic had been perceived by the administration as a slow-moving scientific agency, not as a quick-response organization. Another source of tension could have been that the OWS leadership was intentionally excluding the CDC because of the White House's ire toward Dr. Messonnier—of course undeserved, given that she was indeed right about disruptions to everyday life caused by COVID.

In any public health emergency, it is vital that responsible government officials communicate to the public what is known, what is not known, what is being done to learn more, and what individuals can do to protect themselves and their families.[16] At the beginning of the COVID pandemic, CDC conducted nine media briefings in January and eight in February. But after Dr. Messonnier's remark sparked the president's ire, CDC conducted only two briefings in March 2020, and then none between March 9 and June 12. As congressional investigators later pointed out, over 100,000 Americans died between March 10 and June 12, when the CDC was effectively muzzled by an administration eager to get the economy back to business.[17,18]

The sidelining of the CDC also contributed to a crippling delay in providing useful guidance to the 64 funded state and local immunization program jurisdictions that would be on the front lines coordinating vaccine delivery and administration. The CDC issued its initial planning assumptions to all state and territorial immunization programs on April 23, 2020.[3] The government formally announced the OWS campaign on May 15, 2020.[5] It then took over four months until more comprehensive planning guidance was provided to state and local jurisdictions on September 16, 2020.[19]

This gap is largely attributed to the time it took for CDC to convince OWS leaders of the wisdom to utilize and expand the existing American vaccine distribution system. CDC officials spent months trying to persuade the newly appointed OWS leaders of the soundness of the existing immunization delivery infrastructure and plans, the critical difference between vaccine distribution and vaccine administration, and the need to provide resources to effectively scale up these systems. These efforts were backed up by outreach from national public health organizations directly to OWS leaders. As with other attempts by public health leaders to engage in Trump administration COVID response planning, that outreach was largely ignored.

There were also delays for CDC to get formal approval, or "clearance," to begin a process dubbed "micro-planning." This process was designed to engage state and local officials to build template plans for the coordination of critical state and local vaccine administration activities. CDC officials we interviewed told us that before being allowed to begin the micro-planning process, they first had to answer numerous requests to explain and justify to Army officials every component of their existing immunization delivery infrastructure, including the choice to contract with the private-sector distribution company McKesson. The disagreements early in the planning process reflected both divisions in the details of a preferred approach as well as a clash between the military and public health cultures. As evident from our interviews, these disagreements included utilization of strict chains of command, use of different jargon, preference for different approaches to health care, and dismissal of and lack of respect for women's perspectives.

CDC officials recount being asked for data on certain state and local capacities, such as the number of ultracold freezers available to state and local health departments (author interview with senior CDC official, March 28, 2022). When these officials explained to OWS leaders that it would take a few days to collect that information from the 64 jurisdictions, many of whose staff were helping with other elements of the emergency response before the vaccine became available, the answer was deemed highly unsatisfactory by military officers used to receiving information in real time.

Moreover, it is ironic that while the military is known for its strict chains of command, significant confusion reigned both internally and externally about who was in charge of specific components of the vaccine distribution enterprise. Particularly at CDC, officials told us it was unclear if their staff should report to Secretary Azar or General Perna. Although Secretary Esper was at the top of the chart next to Azar, his role was not clear to outside observers.[7]

Then there was the use of jargon. As one CDC official put it, "Public health does not speak military" (author interview with senior CDC official, March 28, 2022), and certainly the military was unfamiliar with both public health terminology and public health organization. The military is used to a system in which commanding officers have almost complete control over their assigned base, whereas the federalist system of public health in America shares capacity among federal, state, and local health agencies. This decentralized system caused early frustration among General Perna and his staff. As observed by one CDC official:

He's military. So there's one government. He didn't understand, fifty states all have their own opinion . . . Nobody's going to tell them that they need to write a new plan and report to some general they don't know and get ready. And so he immediately wrote them off and said, this is too time consuming to have to talk to fifty governors plus the mayor of New York plus [the other jurisdictions] when I can get the CEOs of CVS and Walgreens on the phone. And we said, "Agreed, welcome to public health." (Author interview with senior CDC official, March 28, 2022.)

In addition, military officers are used to having their commands obeyed rather than questioned or debated by subordinates. But planning for the largest vaccine delivery program in history was unprecedented, with many details worth debating to make sure all contingencies were considered. As the *Washington Post* reported, Dr. Messonnier was known for being plainspoken and "periodically became embroiled in heated arguments with officials from other agencies brought in to assist with the vaccination campaign."[20] The *Post* recounted how after questioning General Perna about distribution during one of the early planning meetings, one of his aides later pulled her aside and said, "That's not how you talk to a four-star general."[20]

Another element of the military and public health culture clash that may have shaded OWS's perspective is the US Army's experience of and approach to health care. As a CDC official we interviewed put it, "In the military you are told what health care you need, where and when you will get it, and then you get it" (author interview with senior CDC official, March 28, 2022). With vaccines for civilians, where consent is based on trust, there is a much greater need to focus on providing clear, fact-based information and generating demand, especially among those who may be hesitant.

CDC officials also reported having to explain why it would be unwise for OWS to circumvent the existing safety review processes run by the Food and Drug Administration (FDA) through its Center for Biologics Evaluation and Research and by the CDC's Advisory Committee on Immunization Practices (ACIP). The attitude of the military, one official said, was that "the vaccine is already paid for. If Pfizer says it's good, why can't we just begin to ship it?" (author interview with senior CDC official, March 28, 2022). While this could be seen as an effort to take the fight to the virus as quickly as possible, it also reflected a critical lack of understanding about the need to build trust among the American people by showing transparently that no corners were being cut in the testing and approval for both safety and effectiveness. Such a move would have won the war more quickly perhaps, but with a tremendous cost to credibly claiming the vaccines were safe and effective.

CDC staff incurred further frustration when they tried to explain to the OWS leadership that waiting the additional 24 to 72 hours for the FDA's and CDC's public advisory committees to meet and make recommendations would be worth the time to help build this public trust. The military mindset, all the way up to the commander in chief, was that there should not be any delays in joining the fight.

Finally, there is the important question about respect for women's opinions among both the military and the core OWS leadership team. In Mango's book,[4] he devotes an entire chapter to describing the extraordinary traits of each member of the core leadership team. These men are described as visionary, brilliant, and egoless team players. It is notable that his only criticisms of personnel are aimed at the two most prominent women in the government's response, Dr. Deborah Birx and Dr. Nancy Messonnier, who were not included in the core OWS leadership team. They are singled out by Mango for harsh criticism for their "style"[4] of presenting their views straightforwardly and for their lack of teamwork. He describes everyone on the all-male OWS board of directors as visionary leaders but ascribes no such traits to the two women involved at the top levels of the effort.

Regardless of the nature of these clashes, the result was an additional delay as CDC waited to receive clearance to issue guidance that was eventually released as the *COVID-19 Vaccination Program Interim Playbook for Jurisdiction Operations* on September 16, nearly six months after OWS was formed and just three months before vaccine deliveries began.[19] Mango continued to be unapologetic about the sidelining of the CDC in the early planning stages.

In addition to complaints about the CDC staff being based in Atlanta, Mango revealed his deep misunderstanding about CDC's capabilities, telling us, "Our assessment of where they were versus where they needed to be to get from point A to point B couldn't have even begun with all the money in the world in the time we had" (author interview with Paul Mango, MBA, December 13, 2021). In the same interview, he continued:

> The CDC is not an operating body. The CDC is an academic institution directly adjacent to the Emory University campus in Atlanta. They are very eager to publish points of view on things. They are not operators. The Army materiel command—they are operators. They understand the intense need for detailed planning. They understand as Gus [Perna] used to call it "the physics of distribution." He used to say at some point our planning is over and it's all about physics. We have to move hundreds of millions of doses from here to here under stringent conditions with no error. CDC had no experience doing that.

Former CDC director Dr. Tom Frieden described the heart of the issue, telling us, "It was very clear that they were really missing the point on distribution. That was a major problem reflecting hubris, reflecting a lack of understanding of public health, and a lack of willingness to listen to public health [experts]" (author interview with Thomas Frieden, MD, June 10, 2022). The result was a mission that was defined too narrowly.

TOP LEADERS DEFINED THE MISSION AND ITS OPERATIONS TOO NARROWLY

With Dr. Messonnier and her team pushed aside, the OWS vaccine distribution team initially moved forward with leaders who had no training in public health or medicine, no understanding of the US public health system, and no understanding of the importance of building trust in vaccines and the behavioral science behind generating demand. It is therefore unsurprising that they initially defined the team's mission as simply delivering the vaccine to the pharmacy or hospital. Journalist Katherine Eban's reporting on the OWS campaign includes mention of a motivational poster placed on an easel outside the door of a conference room used by OWS.[6] It read, "Operation Warp Speed, Winning Matters. Winning 300 Million Doses of Vaccine January 2021."

Further reporting on the culture clash between CDC and OWS leaders, Eban recounts a June 2020 visit CDC staff made to the OWS team in Washington, DC:

> On June 5, a CDC team traveled from its headquarters in Atlanta, Georgia, to Washington, D.C., to brief Operation Warp Speed officials on their view of the essential components of a successful vaccination plan. What they heard back was dismaying. "They told [us] their task was to pick up the vaccine and put it in the trucks and drive it to state health departments and drop it off," said one of the CDC team members.[6]

The team was shocked by the response, which indicated a much narrower understanding of vaccine distribution than what was understood by CDC planners.

Mango attributes this understanding to General Perna's assumption that, as he said, the "physics"[4(p158)] of delivery would take care of everything after that, reflecting a mindset akin to "if we deliver it, they will come." In response, the CDC along with its state and local public health partners spent countless hours during the summer of 2020 trying to help its new Army partners understand the big difference between dropping off vaccines at a state health department and the administration of vaccines to a population. According to Eban's reporting, vaccine expert Dr. Bruce Gellin became concerned about disconnected OWS and CDC perspectives created by OWS operating within a "vaccine world" and CDC operating within a "vaccination world," a disconnect that could create rollout chaos and confusion.[6]

While General Perna brought military precision and vast logistical experience to his role, his lack of public health training or experience led him to define the vaccine delivery mission too narrowly. He partially acknowledged this, introducing himself at a December 2020 White House summit on vaccine distribution by saying, "I am not a scientist, I am a soldier."[21] This limitation was reflected in the two metrics he stressed at that summit, saying that the two key measures for the mission would be, first, the "ability to ship vaccine within 24 hours of the FDA granting emergency use authorization" and, second, "executing a predictable and consistent cadence of vaccine delivery."[21] The number of vaccines administered, however, was not included as a key metric.

No doubt speed of shipping and a predictable delivery are two important measures, but they did not reflect the full complexity of the enterprise nor address issues of expanding provider capacity, determining prioritization, assuring equity, generating demand, reporting data, monitoring coverage and safety, communicating risk and safety, and addressing hesitancy. In short, their two leading metrics stopped at the hospital, clinic, or pharmacy delivery dock and did not extend to what really mattered inside: how many shots got into arms. As Mango told Eban, the OWS leadership's assumptions were "all based on the fundamental belief that local leaders are best positioned to execute. It guided our whole process. We're going to provide you the vaccine for free, all the accoutrements; we are going to distribute to precisely the place you want it; and all you need to do is tell us where."[6] The problem was that delivery and administration, especially with vaccines requiring so many special handling requirements and administration considerations, are inextricably linked.

Public health officials see the vaccine-to-vaccination cycle in distinct stages, including development, production, procurement, distribution, and administration. Often, the term *distribution* is used by some to capture all these phases, not just the discrete process of moving product from manufacturing to a clinical setting. The CDC struggled to convince OWS leaders of the need to focus on the very important details associated with administration and the criticality of last-mile planning and operations—that is, of getting a vaccine out of a box and into an arm at the hyperlocal level. The OWS leaders, by their metrics, did not seem to appreciate why this last mile is so critical and deserved equal attention to that given to vaccine manufacture and procurement.

Indeed, from the start, the political appointees and military leaders of OWS showed little understanding of the existing public-private immunization delivery infrastructure and the need to support the complicated work of getting the shots from the point of vaccine delivery into people's arms. One of the core tenets of the immunization community, attributed to Dr. Walt Orenstein, former director of CDC's National Immunization Program from 1998 to 2004, is "Vaccines don't save lives. Vaccinations save lives."[22] The distinction may not be apparent to people without experience in the field, but it is a critical one. And to people trained in military logistics, not vaccination, it was not immediately understood. In a March 28, 2022, interview with us, one former state health official summarized the critical difference in perspectives: "The one thing I don't think they ever really got, and I still think they don't get, is that the metrics for measuring success is different in logistics than it is in clinical and public health. They look at their measure of success as deliverables and logistically moving vaccine from point A to point B." In this same interview, she continued:

Public health looks at the success rate of administration. How many shots went into arms? That's our measure of how much we succeeded, and they are counter to each other . . . There was never a clear understanding of the two separate and unique matrices that measured success. And there was not a clear understanding from the logistics side of when their job ended. [They thought] their job ended at the point where the vaccine was delivered. "You've got your vaccine, your job is done. A hundred percent of it made it, congratulations, you succeeded." But you need to continue that measurement metric all the way through the delivery into the arm. And now [it may appear you are] wasting vaccine. And they saw that as an interference in their measurable metrics where their role is not part of the administration and clinical process. So that has been a constant misunderstanding that they can't seem to grasp.

The misunderstanding also contributed to the tension around the question of how CDC contributed to or undermined OWS teamwork. Early in his book, Paul Mango says that one of their keys to success was establishing a leadership philosophy that "delegate[ed] key tasks to those who possess the most knowledge or experience . . . [and that] debating differences of opinion was encouraged but [that] undermining the integrity of teamwork was not to be tolerated . . . [and to] rigorously prevent the federal government from engaging in any activities the private sector could perform better."[4(p15)]

By many accounts, Dr. Messonnier, one of the federal officials with the most experience overseeing the distribution of vaccines in America, took advantage of this encouragement to debate differences.[6,20] She and her team tried to convince the OWS core leadership that while there already existed extensive use of private-sector partners in vaccine distribution, including McKesson, and tens of thousands of hospitals, private doctors, clinics, and pharmacies, there were certain activities such as prioritization, enrollment of providers, management and allocation of limited vaccine inventory, and communications that only the public sector could lead.

Her reward for debating differences and forceful advocacy was to be dismissed as "not someone who inspired teamwork and collaboration . . . and entrenched in suspicion of the private sector."[4(p21)] The difficulty she had in representing CDC's perspective, which was truly not that far off from the OWS preference for using the private sector, resulted in great frustration. It again raises the question of whether she would have been listened to were she making the argument as a male military officer rather than as a female medical expert and public health professional. Four months after the vaccine rollout, in April 2021, Dr. Messonnier was "reassigned" to other duties within the CDC. She then took what Biden administration officials stated was an "unplanned vacation" before she ultimately resigned in May 2021.[23]

The OWS concept of operations reflected the enormous logistical resources needed to support the development, manufacture, purchase, and delivery of millions of doses of vaccine. But it also reflected a fundamentally narrow view of the OWS campaign's mission, as it lacked a commensurate focus on the resources needed to administer the vaccine and failed to acknowledge the essential role of state and local public health agencies in turning vaccines into vaccinations. For example, vaccines cannot simply be delivered to providers. While seemingly bureaucratic, each provider site needed to sign an enrollment agreement with the government committing to proper vaccine storage, to administer the vaccine in accordance with CDC recommendations, and to report on all administered doses within 72 hours—all this for legal reasons and patient protections. Because eventually tens of thousands of such sites were enrolled, the federal government could in no way have the capacity to oversee such an enterprise.

This labor-intensive work fell to the state and local jurisdictions. Robert Swanson, former immunization program manager for Michigan, described the pressure this placed on states:

> Everybody wanted the vaccine at the beginning, but we had to go out and assess were they ready to receive the vaccine. We had to train them on proper storage and handling and administration of the vaccine. And then there's the standpoint of just coordinating all the different types of health care providers in the state. One staff member was the lead working with pharmacists, one was lead with private docs—many of which couldn't get the vaccine right away at all. And then obviously the big hospitals and trying to get it out equitably to them. It was just a tremendous amount of work. (Author interview with Robert Swanson, MPH, January 10, 2022.)

But the early OWS planning reflected a military mindset that conceived of the operation's role as limited to delivering the vaccine and that expected the administration would somehow take care of itself. Again, an "if you build it, they will come" and "physics will take over" mentality seriously underestimated what it takes to move the vaccine the last mile from its delivery point and into people's arms.

DELAYED ENGAGEMENT WITH STATE AND LOCAL PUBLIC HEALTH LEADERS

As described in Chapter 2, on June 23, 2020, the leaders of the key associations representing state and local public health officials and immunization program managers sent a letter to General Perna and Dr. Slaoui offering support, sharing initial recommendations, and posing key questions about the vaccine development process. The letter also asked for dialogue and underscored the need for close cooperation with state, territorial, tribal, and local public health agencies and immunization programs. As noted, the OWS leadership never acknowledged the outreach although contact was eventually made with subordinates. And while the top OWS leaders had some ad hoc regional calls with various state health leaders, they never met with or spoke directly with the leadership of the national organizations most directly involved in the state and local vaccine distribution enterprise to discuss planning assumptions and considerations.

This was a missed opportunity for OWS leaders. One of the greatest benefits of working through national associations representing states is that they can provide a forum to reach all states and territories at one time rather than having 50 separate conversations with each state, or the 64 state, territorial, District of Columbia, freely associated state, and local jurisdictions in the case of CDC-funded immunization programs. These associations can also canvas their entire membership to help distill the common questions and concerns shared by all jurisdictions as well as the unique challenges limited to a particular state or region. In essence, they offer the best mechanism to ensure close coordination between federal, state, and local governments.

By nature of partially funding this infrastructure, CDC is aware of the value in working through national groups of public health professionals. But despite the apparent urging by CDC to utilize this network, OWS core leadership did not heed the CDC's advice. Accordingly, these groups were never asked for input into the emerging federal plan nor allowed to provide feedback once it was drafted. There were never any conversations about coordinating key messages among federal, state, and local spokespersons. Most important, OWS leaders never asked frontline immunization program managers for their professional judgment on the resources needed to adequately support the state and local response. Instead, they actively tried to convince states that they did not need the resources they were requesting. There was a belief that the strong partnership between CDC and state health leaders built over years of collaboration and public health emergency responses was just a "mutual admiration society"[4(p109)] and not an effective mechanism for communication, information sharing, situational awareness, and implementation planning.

States in turn were trying desperately to educate the OWS team on the importance of core state activities that were critical to the last mile leading up to vaccine administration. These activities include enrolling providers, operating data systems to collect and analyze information on every dose delivered and administered, managing inventory, assuring that vaccine is being shipped equitably to every community, and assuring availability of centralized appointment-scheduling systems.

For months, CDC leaders pressed OWS on the need to engage routinely with state and public health officials to ensure coordination and avoid some of the crucial mistakes observed in earlier pandemic responses, including the response to H1N1. Finally, after a three-month delay, in mid-August 2020, CDC was finally given clearance to begin a process to engage states in micro-planning. Teams from CDC, DoD, and the Indian Health Service initially visited sites in North Dakota and Florida and engaged virtually with California, Minnesota, and Philadelphia. There were five objectives of micro-planning[24]:

1. Accelerate state, local, and tribal readiness for a large-scale vaccination campaign;
2. Better inform OWS understanding of jurisdiction plans and technical assistance needs;
3. Provide technical assistance to jurisdictions on their COVID-19 vaccine planning process;

4. Develop model plans to be shared with all jurisdictions before COVID-19 vaccine release; and

5. Build on expanded influenza vaccination campaign planning work.

How seriously the state input into micro-planning was taken remains unclear, but it did serve the purpose of beginning to convince OWS leaders of the central importance of state and local health departments. Maybe there was more value to a strong federal-state partnership than mutual admiration after all. One state official we interviewed recounted the sense that the CDC officials involved in the jurisdictional meetings would ask questions whose answers they wanted their OWS colleagues to hear—namely, the recommendations CDC had been telling them all along—but they wanted OWS leaders to hear them directly from the states.

By September, the OWS brass began to warm up to partnerships with states. A strategy overview issued by HHS and DoD concurrent with the release of the *CDC Playbook* on September 16, 2020, entitled *From the Factory to the Frontlines*, laid out four tasks necessary for the COVID-19 vaccine program, with the very first being to "engage with state, tribal, territorial, and local partners, other stakeholders, and the public to communicate public health information around the vaccine and promote vaccine confidence and uptake."[25(p2)]

Later, at a December 8, 2020, White House summit, Paul Mango described the OWS "partnership principle" as "federally supported, state-managed, and locally executed."[21] That same day, General Perna said that one of the keys to their success would be their approach: "It's not our plan that needs to be implemented perfectly, it's the Governors' plans that we want to empower and enable. We want to make sure we execute according to their priorities. They know their states, they know their people. Our position is to empower them."[21] But the core OWS leadership's depth of misunderstanding about the role of states was revealed just days after the White House summit in an interview Paul Mango conducted with the Pittsburgh Technology Council on December 21, 2020, at which he stated:

> Because the states . . . The only thing they really have to do is tell us where they want things shipped and everything is shipped there. The vaccines, the needles, the syringes, the swabs, the face masks, dry ice, even, we're even shipping out dry ice, and we'll ship to any corner of Fifth and Vine in the country. Just tell us where to get it. So . . . I think they're going to be using a lot of those funds for maybe some advertising and to address vaccine hesitancy and those types of things.[26]

That as late in the planning as December 3, 2020, Mango believed the campaign would be a "mop-up" operation by the end of January underscores the significant misunderstanding of the vaccine distribution and administration effort.[2] More important, however, is that the OWS leadership had for months been undermining their prospects for a smooth vaccine rollout by delaying guidance to state immunization programs and actively lobbying against additional congressional appropriations to fund state and local vaccine distribution and administration.

BLOCKING RESOURCES FOR THE LAST MILE

In a national interview broadcast on C-SPAN commemorating the anniversary of the first COVID shot being administered, Paul Mango stated that OWS had spent $30 billion by the time the Trump administration left office on January 20, 2021.[27] Of that amount, HHS had initially directed a paltry $200 million to state and territorial health departments to prepare for COVID vaccine delivery, and this was not approved until September 23, 2020.[28] An additional $140 million was awarded in December 2020, almost at the same time vaccine shipments began. This represented about $1 per American to prepare for the most complicated and important vaccine distribution program in US history. In contrast, a coalition of state and local public health associations led by the Association of State and Territorial Health Officials (ASTHO) and Association of Immunization Managers (AIM) estimated that at least $8.4 billion would be needed for successful state and local vaccination distribution and administration activities.

Work to develop an estimate of how much it would cost to vaccinate the entire nation began in April 2020. Because it had never been done before, there was no existing model to utilize. Staff from AIM and ASTHO began by examining estimates and actual costs encountered in the 2009 H1N1 influenza vaccine campaign. Using H1N1 distribution expenditures as a baseline and factoring for inflation, staff began to consider the unique factors to take into account to successfully vaccinate nearly the entire American public with a novel vaccine. During the H1N1 influenza pandemic from June 2009 through December 2010, HHS spent $4.17 billion from a 2009 supplemental appropriation, according to the agency's reports to Congress.[29] Of the $4.17 billion spent by HHS, about $1.72 billion (41%) was spent on vaccine production, including the purchase of the H1N1 vaccine, as well as adjuvants and supplies such as needles and syringes, to be distributed along with the H1N1 vaccine.[30] HHS specifically purchased over 190 million doses of the H1N1 vaccine and 200 million ancillary supply kits. Approximately $1.49 billion (36%) was spent to support state and local response; most of these funds were provided to the states through Public Health Emergency Response grants. In addition, approximately $340 million was dedicated to the CDC vaccination campaign, including contracts to support vaccine distribution, vaccine safety and effectiveness monitoring, and a communications campaign on vaccination and prevention.

With these resources, CDC estimated that from October 2009 through May 2010, 81 million people were vaccinated against H1N1 influenza (27% of the US population over the age of six months), including about 34% of individuals in the initial target groups.[29] This represented just one-fourth of the total US population in 2020. In addition, the H1N1 vaccine required only one dose, while initial planning assumptions for the COVID vaccine already anticipated that at least two doses would be needed. So, while the amount spent on the H1N1 vaccine provided a baseline, it was clear the scope and other anticipated challenges would require additional resources.

Concurrent to the initial explorations to develop a funding estimate for a national COVID vaccine distribution effort, in April 2020 Congress was continuing to consider supplemental emergency requests. With so many unknowns so early in the pandemic, it was difficult to develop even a credible ballpark estimate. Nonetheless, on April 9, 2020, AIM issued a statement urging Congress to invest in three key areas to strengthen the nation's immunization infrastructure to prepare for mass vaccination against COVID-19: (1) immunization information systems, (2) staffing, and (3) outreach and communication.[31] The statement did not include any specific dollar amounts but did set the tone for the challenge ahead. Michele Roberts, the immunization program manager in Washington and then chair of the AIM Executive Committee, said, "Once a COVID-19 vaccine is available, it will be all-hands-on-deck. We save lives with vaccines every day, but this is an unprecedented opportunity to protect American lives. With immediate investment and focused preparation, we hope to protect all Americans from COVID-19."[31]

During this nascent planning in the spring of 2020, the US Congress passed the first of five emergency supplemental funding bills. The Coronavirus Preparedness and Response Supplemental Appropriations Act was passed with near-unanimous support and was signed into law by President Trump on March 6, 2020. The bill provided $8.3 billion in emergency funding for federal agencies to respond to the coronavirus outbreak, including more than $3 billion for research and development of vaccines, therapeutics, and diagnostics to prevent or treat the effects of coronavirus.[32] Understandably, the primary focus at this point in the pandemic was on vaccine development, not distribution and administration. Nevertheless, this bill provided no funds to support state planning and infrastructure improvements needed for vaccine distribution and administration, despite being a reasonably foreseeable need at that time.

Congress passed three additional supplemental spending bills in March and April 2020, but again these bills included funds only for vaccine research, development, manufacture, and purchase, not for distribution.[33] As spring turned to summer, Senator Patty Murray (D-WA), then ranking member of the Senate Health, Education, Labor, and Pensions Committee, on July 13, 2020, released a comprehensive plan entitled *The Democratic COVID-19 Response: A Roadmap to Getting a Safe and Effective Vaccine to All.*[34] Despite the title reflecting the unfortunate partisan framing of the pandemic, the centerpiece of the plan stated, "Congress should provide $25 billion in new emergency funding to support additional research and development, manufacturing, purchase, distribution, and administration of COVID-19 vaccines."[34] In addition, Topher Spiro and Dr. Ezekiel (Zeke) Emanuel, two leading experts in government and public health then with the

Center for American Progress, released a report near the end of July entitled *A Comprehensive COVID-19 Vaccine Plan: Efficient Manufacturing, Financing, and Distribution of a COVID-19 Vaccine.*[35] Their plan estimated that a total of close to $40.6 billion would be needed to support the full range of vaccine manufacturing, purchase, and distribution. The plan included $10 billion to support vaccine operations at community clinics, $1.5 billion to cover the cost of vaccinating the uninsured, and notably, $7.2 billion to support global vaccine efforts.

Throughout the summer of 2020, Congress was stuck in negotiations to develop an additional COVID aid package. While prior congressional action had provided the money OWS was using to speed up the vaccine development and manufacturing process, Congress had still not allocated any additional funds specifically for vaccine delivery and administration.

To address this growing concern, AIM released a statement in early September, declaring:

> Substantial resources are needed to implement state plans and ensure that cost is not a barrier to any American receiving COVID-19 vaccine. AIM reiterates its call for Congress to include an adequate appropriation in a COVID-19 relief bill or funding agreement in the coming weeks. To date, Congress has not authorized any explicit funding for the critical vaccine distribution activities that need to happen in every community across the nation. Funding only vaccine development without providing adequate resources for distribution, tracking, and monitoring would be tragic.[30]

The AIM statement laid out a series of specific activities that would need to be undertaken by state and local public health agencies, including these:

- Recruiting and training the necessary additional workforce for the state, local, tribal, and territorial health departments; primary care settings; and pharmacies—with special focus on reaching communities of color and other vulnerable populations;
- Planning to stand-up supplemental vaccination sites and promote new strategies for mass vaccination, such as drive-thru clinics and clinics in nontraditional locations that are easy to access and are safe for vaccinators and the public;
- Enhancing existing public health infrastructure and adapting immunization information systems—where appropriate—to meet emerging data standards;
- Strengthening vaccine confidence and combating misinformation with federally supported and locally tailored communication, research, and outreach efforts;
- Developing and distributing tools and resources for health care providers prior to the administration of COVID-19 vaccines;
- Purchasing any necessary personal protective equipment for vaccinators that is not supplied by the federal government; and
- Concurrently supporting influenza vaccination campaigns and other routine immunizations.

Reflecting the urgency of the situation, Claire Hannan said at that time:

> Time is of the essence—we urge Congress to find bipartisan agreement on vaccine distribution resources as soon as possible. There are many challenges ahead. No one expects this will be easy, but my entire experience in public health has shown that the people dedicated to protecting and saving the lives of people they have never even met will find a way to get this done. We have the opportunity to put together a plan now that can help end this pandemic. We can't afford not to invest in that; and we cannot fail because the lives of our neighbors and the livelihood of our neighborhoods are at stake. A national COVID-19 vaccination program should go down in history as the greatest public health operation of our generation.[30]

A week later, on September 16, 2020, CDC director Dr. Robert Redfield appeared at a hearing before the US Senate Appropriations Committee Health Subcommittee. Dr. Redfield made no request for vaccine distribution resources in his prepared remarks.[36] However, in response to a question from the committee chair, Senator Roy Blunt (R-MO), Dr. Redfield stated, "We need to get resources to states now. They cannot do it without resources. In my professional opinion . . . it's going to take somewhere between $5.5 to $6 billion to distribute this vaccine. It's as urgent as getting these manufacturing facilities up."[19,37] Senator Blunt, a member of the GOP leadership, replied, "If you have the vaccine and don't have either the plan or the resources to distribute it, that's a huge failure on the part of Congress."[37]

Despite the professional judgment of the CDC director and the concurrence of a key Republican Senate leader, in the weeks and months following this public exchange, Paul Mango began a lobbying campaign against the very resources the CDC would need to support vaccine distribution partners in states. *STAT News* later broke the story of how Mango unapologetically lobbied against HHS's state and local partners, telling congressional aides on October 27, 2020, that states did not need additional funds because they had not yet fully spent the $200 million in planning funds announced just 37 days earlier.[38] When asked what information Paul Mango had that gave him confidence to overrule his own department's CDC director, Mango again displayed his lack of support for state and local public health agencies, telling us:

> Part of it was economic—they [CDC] asked for multiple billions of dollars to give to the public health agencies so they could do this. We were, like, Wait a minute. The vaccine is free. All the ancillary supplies—the syringes and needles—are free. The federal government is going to reimburse providers $28 per injection, commercial insurers even more than that . . . Why do you need this $5 or $6 billion for the public health agencies? Plus we were going to be a little constrained for procurement, because remember the supplemental to the CARES Act didn't pass until December. So all fall we were scrounging . . . So they wanted a bunch of money to send down to the public health agencies and we were, like, "For what?" (author interview with Paul Mango, MBA, December 13, 2021)

The "what" that state and local public agencies were expected to do was explained first in an August 4, 2020, CDC letter to states that included a checklist of activities for states and jurisdictions to guide accelerated planning.[39] It directed states to conduct a series of prioritized vaccination planning efforts, including convening a planning team, identifying critical occupational groups likely to be prioritized for initial doses, planning for temporary mass vaccination clinics, augmenting existing capacity, identifying areas in need of additional outreach, and preparing information systems to meet forthcoming data standards.

The August letter was the first real guidance state and local jurisdictions had received since April. This checklist was expanded and formalized when CDC and HHS released the operational *CDC Playbook* on September 16, 2020.[19] Playbook guidance outlined six main areas where states would play a lead role: (1) providing outreach and education to critical populations; (2) recruiting, enrolling, and training vaccine providers; (3) overseeing vaccine ordering, distribution, and inventory management; (4) documenting vaccine administration and reporting via immunization information systems; (5) leading state-based communications; and (6) collaborating on safety monitoring.[19] It is important to note that states were undertaking all this planning activity still not knowing which vaccines would be authorized or what their storage and dosing requirements would be, among many other unknowns in the nascent process.

The lack of serious consideration of resources needed by state and local jurisdictions was exasperating to state and local officials. It was as if the commanders in Washington were sending their troops into battle without listening to what they said they needed to win. Nevertheless, despite the detailed state expectations laid out in the CDC guidance, Mango told congressional appropriations staff that the money Redfield requested was not needed, according to reporting by *STAT News*'s Nikolas Florko. Florko reported that Mango told him that Redfield's 2020 request was "lobbying Congress for money behind our back."[38] "I call it the mutual-admiration society—they were trying to help their friends at the state public health offices even though they didn't have any real plan to spend the money,"[38] Mango said in the interview, seeming again to indicate that having professional rapport and respect between federal and state officials is somehow a bad thing and ignoring the myriad expectations laid out for jurisdictions in the playbook.

Beyond that judgment, Mango also indicated his opposition was founded on reports that states had not yet drawn down the $200 million in planning grants and they had not provided adequate "business plans." *STAT News* reported that Mango told Congress, "If we get those things, we will be the first to let you know and we will be happy to give them more money."[38]

Later, to ward off further misperceptions that states were not spending federal dollars to support the vaccination campaign, ASTHO and AIM wrote a memo to senior HHS officials on December 4, 2020, providing several reasons why the money was not appearing in the HHS financial reporting system as spent.[40] First, the $200 million was announced only weeks earlier, on September 20, 2020, and the tracking of government expenditures often suffers from a significant reporting lag. Second, many states made plans to obligate their available funds but needed time to execute contracts with their local partners. Third, states reported that they were hesitant to hire additional staff with a one-time emergency allocation, thereby acknowledging the difficulty in recruiting qualified staff without any assurance of job security. Fourth, at the time of these awards, there was no indication that any additional funds would be available in the future, so some states reported a desire to hold the money in reserve until actual vaccinations began and spend other emergency supplemental appropriations first. Finally, the organizations noted the delays in the time money was obligated compared to the time it showed up in the HHS systems as expended. The memo concluded:

> For these reasons, spenddown is not the correct metric of current and future need for resources. Instead, federal officials should work directly with the federal and state technical monitors and program officers for each state's vaccination program and discuss spend plans with state and territorial health officials and Governor's offices to better understand the planned expenditures and activities accomplished to date to assess what resources may be needed in the future.
>
> Additionally, HHS should consider that there are activities that will be required in every state and territory that are not reimbursable to an insurance program, public fund for health care, or to be provided by federal agencies and contractors.[40]

While all these are reasonable explanations, HHS never did engage in dialogue with state officials to ask why the data they had on the pace of drawdown was slow. In fact, in October, after Secretary Azar publicly stated that states did not need any more resources for vaccine distribution and administration, leaders from ASTHO and AIM sent him a letter asking for a meeting to discuss state needs and the rationale for more resources. Continuing the long tradition of senior Trump officials refusing to speak directly with state public health leaders before setting policy, the meeting request was acknowledged but declined on behalf of Secretary Azar by the HHS Office of Intergovernmental Affairs.

White House and HHS officials also said that their opposition to more funding was founded on the lack of state business plans to spend the money. However, HHS at no point ever asked the states to provide a budget or estimate resource needs. The CDC said states and jurisdictions should use the interim playbook to develop and update their COVID-19 vaccination plans, but nowhere in the guidance were jurisdictions requested to provide a budget for those activities. The word *budget* does not appear anywhere in the federal document. Some states even remarked at the time that developing a vaccine distribution plan divorced from a budget was more akin to developing a wish list. Yet, the administration was in effect dinging states for not providing spending plans that were never asked for. Mango's insistence that distribution activities were already paid for indicates quite the opposite, as described in the initial memo sent by ASTHO, AIM, the National Association of County and City Health Officials (NACCHO), and the American Immunization Registry Association to OWS that summer.

When CDC sought the resources necessary to scale up and support state and local public health agencies, it was Paul Mango who stood in the way. So, the question needs to be asked, Why would the self-described foremost leader of the OWS campaign be so adamantly opposed to providing resources to state and local public health agencies? His book reveals some answers. In it, Mango recounts how Secretary Azar told their private-sector partners to "plan as if they were limited only by science and physics"—in other words, do not worry about the money HHS would supply.[4(p28)] Mango also asserts that the economic return from the government's investment in vaccine development was nearly infinite. But this generosity with taxpayer funds did not extend to the public-sector partners in the enterprise. Mango takes credit for overruling the CDC's $6 billion budget request and particularly belittles a line it proposed asking for $1 billion for "unforeseen contingencies." He describes this as "the last straw" and unacceptable use of taxpayer dollars.[4(p108)] Money was available for private-sector work, but not for the governmental public health agencies accountable to their citizens for providing them with vaccinations.

It is a surprising objection coming from a West Point graduate who should be familiar with General Dwight Eisenhower's famous maxim about planning for contingencies. In a 1957 speech, then-president Eisenhower said, "Plans are worthless, but planning is everything. There is a very great distinction because when you are planning for an emergency you must start with this one thing: the very definition of 'emergency' is that it is unexpected, therefore it is not going to happen the way you are planning."[41] The concept is similar to an adage attributed to a Prussian military commander who reportedly said, "No plan survives first contact with the enemy," or the more modern adaptation espoused by boxer Mike Tyson that "everybody has a plan until they get punched in the mouth."[42] After being punched by two major virus variants, the need to address rampant misinformation and deeply entrenched vaccine hesitancy, and unexpected recommendations for booster shots, CDC's contingencies request that Mango described as the last straw certainly seems prescient.

Although it was too late to be effective in being adequately prepared when vaccines were first rolled out at the state and local levels, Congress in essence overruled the administration's opposition to state and local vaccine distribution funding and, after months of delay, specifically directed billions toward vaccine distribution funding in a massive relief package signed into law on December 28, 2020. The law included $8.75 billion "to plan, prepare for, promote, distribute, administer, monitor, and track coronavirus vaccines to ensure broad-based distribution, access, and vaccine coverage."[43(p731)] Of this amount, Congress specified that $4.5 billion was to be directed to state, local, territorial, and tribal public health departments, with $1 billion to be sent out within

21 days of enactment. The law also included $300 million for a targeted effort to distribute and administer vaccines to high-risk and underserved populations, including racial and ethnic minority populations and rural communities. Finally, the law required that the CDC

> develop a comprehensive coronavirus vaccine distribution strategy and spend plan, including how existing infrastructure will be leveraged, enhancements or new infrastructure that may be built, considerations for moving and storing vaccines, guidance for how governmental public health entities should prepare for, store, and administer vaccines, nationwide vaccination targets, funding that will be distributed to states, localities, and territories, how an informational campaign to inform both the public and health care providers will be executed, and how the strategy and plan will focus efforts on high-risk and underserved populations, including racial and ethnic minority populations.[43(p732)]

These are all critical considerations and directives. They just came six months too late to be effective in the critical early days of the vaccine rollout.

LACK OF RESPECT FOR CAREER PUBLIC HEALTH OFFICIALS

In the end, it is almost surprising how well the vaccine rollout worked, considering the seemingly unnecessary tensions encountered in the planning process. Officials from the CDC were not included on the core OWS leadership team and were excluded from early decision-making. Ultimately, OWS leaders largely adopted the vaccine distribution plan that the CDC was already developing when the US Army was inserted into the process.

The initial CDC planning memo issued in April 2020, for example, included a set of planning assumptions that almost completely turned out to be correct.[3] While indicating the CDC plan was to build upon earlier pandemic planning, CDC officials noted that the etiology of COVID was different from that of influenza and plans could change, but they offered the following guidance:

- Limited COVID-19 vaccine doses may be available as early as fall, 2020.
- Initial COVID-19 vaccination efforts should target those in the critical workforce who provide health care and maintain essential functions of society, and then those at highest risk developing complications from COVID-19, depending on supply.
- Initial doses of COVID-19 vaccine may be authorized for use under an Emergency Use Authorization (EUA) issued by the Food and Drug Administration (FDA), based upon available safety and efficacy data.
- Two doses of pandemic COVID-19 vaccine, separated by ≥28 days, may be needed for immunity, requiring the ability to track vaccination administration and provide patient reminders.
- Routine immunization programs will continue.

- Recommendations on groups to target will likely change throughout the response, depending on vaccine supply and disease epidemiology.
- Public demand for COVID-19 vaccination will likely be high, especially when there is limited supply and if there is severe disease in the community.
- Seasonal influenza vaccination will be particularly important for all persons ≥6 months of age, especially front-line HCPs, to limit influenza as another respiratory illness.
- Assuming COVID-19 will continue to spread in the community in the fall and next year, vaccination plans must ensure vaccine clinics will not put patients at risk for COVID-19, which in the setting of mass vaccination may need to include considerations for personal protective equipment (PPE), social distancing or spacing of persons vaccinated and staff, and scheduling individual vaccination appointment times, among other approaches.
- IIS [Immunization Information Systems] will be used to document vaccination and mass-vaccination modules in IIS may be needed, in addition, CDC is exploring additional systems and tools for targeting and tracking vaccination of critical workforce.[3]

While the memo correctly predicted that initial demand for vaccines would be high, it did not mention the need for planning to address specific communities and populations where vaccine demand could be predictably low. It also did not anticipate at that time the possible need for ultracold storage of at least one of the vaccine candidates. These cold chain storage and handling requirements would emerge as one of the most unique challenges in the enterprise.

Nevertheless, the memo confirmed that the nation should be building upon the existing distribution system on which state and local programs had successfully partnered for decades, stating that "CDC currently assumes COVID-19 vaccine distribution and tracking will be conducted using principles exercised in influenza pandemic planning."[3] One of these core principles and pillars of the existing CDC vaccine distribution system is that publicly financed vaccines are distributed through a private-sector pharmaceutical shipping company (McKesson) to largely private-sector providers known as points of care where the vaccine is administered. These points of care include pharmacies, long-term care settings, the Indian Health Service, other federal entity sites, hospitals, doctors' clinics, mobile vaccination sites, schools, and, as a safety net where no other capacity exists, local health departments.[19] This was almost exactly the approach adopted by OWS after months of delay.

The April 2020 CDC planning assumptions also hinted that the scale of the crisis would require enrollment of many additional points of care, maintaining that "when COVID-19 vaccine becomes available, distribution will be through existing infrastructure used for publicly funded routine vaccines. Distribution may be expanded to include additional health care organizations and vaccination providers who can provide pandemic vaccinations to targeted groups."[3] At that time, over 44,000 mostly private-sector health care providers were already enrolled in the VFC program operated jointly by CDC and the states. But since children under age 18 represent only 22% of the population, it was clear from the start that tens of thousands of additional providers would need to be enrolled to reach the entire adult population. Also clear was that special attention would be needed to reach the close to two million residents of nursing homes and other long-term care facilities where many of those most vulnerable to COVID lived.

A precedent for CDC and state immunization programs to rapidly scale up beyond VFC's pediatric capacity to meet increased vaccine demand had been set during the 2009 H1N1 influenza pandemic. The biggest adjustment needed, then, was the inclusion of non-VFC providers such as retail pharmacies, corporations with occupational health clinics, and nonpediatric health care providers as critical vaccine administrators.[44] These types of providers were critical in administering 80 million doses of influenza vaccine in 2009 and would be even more critical in the national campaign to administer any eventual COVID vaccine.

In addition to requiring these private providers, the CDC advocated for continued use of McKesson Corporation as the central vaccine distributor. Along with the many private-sector partners involved in the COVID vaccine distribution enterprise, McKesson deserves special mention for the experience and dedication its team brought to the effort. In the simplest terms, the vaccine distribution CDC proposed to OWS built upon the process already in place for the VFC program. The CDC makes allocations of vaccine to the states, orders are placed by providers to the states via a system called VTrckS, the CDC aggregates the orders and sends them to McKesson, and McKesson picks, packs, and ships the orders to the specified sites, maintaining cold chain integrity throughout the process.[45]

As such, it is baffling that Paul Mango's history of OWS notes that one of the central tensions stemmed from an Army Materiel Command and CDC "debate on whether public health agencies or the private sector would take over vaccine distribution."[4] From the CDC's perspective, though a public-sector agency, it had for decades been using a private-sector distributor, McKesson, to deliver vaccines largely through private-sector health care providers. Nevertheless, Mango reports otherwise in his book:

> Dr. Messonnier had a strong preference for using the nation's public health agencies to both distribute and administer the vaccine doses. The Army team, led by Gen. Gus Perna, which had been supporting combat operations in the Middle East for nearly two decades, had a strong preference for using the more nimble, innovative private sector partners for these tasks. We eventually chose the private sector, and these partners wound up performing their tasks nearly flawlessly.[4(p20)]

Why would the man who describes himself as the foremost leader of OWS so erroneously characterize the CDC's position? Is it possible he did not understand what the CDC was already doing to distribute publicly financed vaccines through the

VFC program? Did Dr. Messonnier and other CDC officials simply not communicate clearly how the existing US vaccine distribution system extensively utilized private-sector partners? The answer is partially revealed in Paul Mango's book and interviews about it.

Mango provides a lively accounting of Secretary Azar's vision to galvanize a public-private partnership whose achievement rightly stands next to other quintessential governmental achievements like the Manhattan Project and the Apollo moon landing. He describes the extraordinary leadership that Moncef Slaoui and Gus Perna brought to the effort and establishes without question that success could not have happened without them. The book also provides a cogent recounting of key lessons learned and gives credit to General Perna and the military leaders from the Army Materiel Command. But in giving nearly all the credit to the US Army and barely acknowledging the critical contributions of thousands of dedicated public health officials at the federal, state, and local levels, Mango provides an incomplete version of the operation. Despite quoting Dr. Slaoui as saying his *modus operandi* is to "give others credit," Mango for some reason does not see fit to give credit to both the Army and the CDC.[4]

Yes, the leadership the OWS team provided was extraordinary, even unprecedented, and it deserves to be celebrated as the great American achievement that it is. Bringing a safe and effective vaccine to market in record time could not have happened without them. There is no way the Biden administration could have ramped up the pace of vaccinations without the solid foundation built by OWS in the months prior to Biden's election. But in essence Mango describes a public-private partnership that at every turn minimizes the vital role of the public sector. Mango should not take away from OWL's achievement but rather provide a more balanced and fuller historical account and avoid mischaracterizations and omissions.

Specifically, Mango mischaracterizes the capacity and positions advocated by the CDC and fails to recognize the critical role played by state and local public health agencies. In book interviews, he makes clear that this refusal to acknowledge the critical contributions of federal, state, and local public health agencies resulted from the OWS leadership team's philosophy that "had an inveterate belief in the private sector *over* the public sector [emphasis added]."[46]

The first red flag appears in the book's subtitle. Released at a time when nearly 1,000 Americans were still dying every day and the nation was approaching one million COVID deaths, nearly half of them after a safe, effective, and free vaccine became widely available, the author's inclusion of the phrase "Inside the Operation That *Beat COVID* [emphasis added]"[4] in the subtitle reflects a certain hubris and lack of empathy. It also echoes the public relations debacle of President George W. Bush's declaration of the end of combat operations in Iraq under a "Mission Accomplished" banner. Another red flag is Mango's assertion in interviews that his is "not a political book."[4] This, however, is belied by the obvious fact that Paul Mango was a political appointee of President Donald

Trump, and the book begins with a foreword by Republican US senator and potential presidential contender Tom Cotton (R-AR).

It seems an odd choice to begin a nonpolitical book with a message from a politician, whose message sets a decidedly political tone. Senator Cotton praises Paul Mango's leadership while assailing the "public health bureaucracy," disparaging "experts" because of their "sheer number of mistakes and inaccurate predictions."[4(p7)] Senator Cotton continues, "Despite their overweening self-confidence and self-regard, the public health 'experts' seemed to get everything wrong." It is interesting that Senator Cotton fails to mention that he is the son of two career bureaucrats: his mother a teacher and middle school principal and his father a retired field supervisor for the Arkansas Department of Public Health.[47]

The perplexing message from Senator Cotton's introduction essentially says you can't trust the public health experts (who are on the frontiers of science dealing with a previously unknown virus), but you can trust my friend Paul Mango. But what is missing in Mango's story is any adequate acknowledgment of the critical contributions made by the public sector—by health officials from the CDC and state and local health departments. Whether you like experts or not, advocacy experts lobbied Congress for the resources needed for the entire enterprise, scientific experts developed the vaccine, military experts helped deliver it, and public health and medical experts administered it.

LEARNING FOR THE NEXT PANDEMIC

The OWS campaign was a tremendous success for several reasons, but it also created significant challenges for public health agencies as they prepared to vaccinate the nation. The sidelining of public health experts, the minimization of state and territorial health agency needs for vaccine distribution and administration, and the disdain for public-sector contributions to the effort were unnecessary and demoralizing at a time when public health was doing everything possible to contain and mitigate the threat posed by COVID. Our criticisms of OWS and its leaders are meant, not to tarnish the operation's achievements, but rather to tell a more complete, and in our view more accurate, story of its game-changing effort as well as the cost of the effort on others.

The five challenges that we have described in this chapter should not be repeated in future efforts to confront a novel pandemic virus. Instead, anticipating and remediating each in future planning and response efforts can only enhance the effectiveness of what comes next. But what would this look like in practice?

First, any effort to rapidly develop a vaccine to end a pandemic should include those agencies that are going to administer the final product from the very beginning of the effort, not the end of it. Even in an emergency, collaboration and partnership are vital to building trust and for including the expertise needed to solve vexing problems.

Second, focusing on vaccine development and production without a commensurate focus on its administration, including addressing hesitancy and concerns about safety, is a huge mistake. Just as important as developing a vaccine is making sure everything possible is done at the outset of development to turn the vaccine into a vaccination.

Third, failing to build upon the existing vaccine infrastructure in initial planning assumptions leads to wasted effort and redundancies. The goal of future campaigns should be to continuously build upon what works and scale systems in place beforehand rather than create new, and untested, processes.

Fourth, while investments in the private sector can yield tremendous results, investments in the public sector are equally important to delivering value to stakeholders and to the communities to which they are accountable.

Finally, respect for expertise and acknowledging the contributions of diverse perspectives in any future campaign are paramount to assuring the best possible result with the least possible harm to others. As described in the next chapter, there were numerous variables, contingencies, and details that planners had to confront in planning the COVID vaccination campaign. All these thousand details could have been dealt with much more effectively in a context of collaboration and partnership rather than disdain and dismissiveness.

REFERENCES

1. National Archives and Records Administration. Remarks by President Trump at the Operation Warp Speed Vaccine Summit. December 8, 2020. Available at: https://trumpwhitehouse.archives.gov/briefings-statements/remarks-president-trump-operation-warp-speed-vaccine-summit. Accessed September 11, 2022.
2. Diamond D. The crash landing of "Operation Warp Speed." *Politico*. January 17, 2021. Available at: https://www.politico.com/news/2021/01/17/crash-landing-of-operation-warp-speed-459892. Accessed September 11, 2022.
3. Centers for Disease Control and Prevention. COVID-19 pandemic vaccination planning: high-level overview for state and local public health programs, April 22, 2020, Letter to States.
4. Mango P. *Warp Speed: Inside the Operation That Beat COVID, the Critics, and the Odds*. New York, NY: Republic Book Publishers; 2022.
5. National Archives and Records Administration. Remarks by President Trump on vaccine development. May 15, 2020. Available at: https://trumpwhitehouse.archives.gov/briefings-statements/remarks-president-trump-vaccine-development. Accessed September 11, 2022.
6. Eban K. "A huge potential for chaos": how the COVID-19 vaccine rollout was hobbled by turf wars and magical thinking. *Vanity Fair*. February 5, 2021. Available at: https://www.vanityfair.com/news/2021/02/how-the-covid-19-vaccine-rollout-was-hobbled. Accessed September 12, 2022.
7. Florko N. New document reveals scope and structure of Operation Warp Speed and underscores vast military involvement. *STAT*. September 28, 2020. Available at: https://www.statnews.com/2020/09/28/operation-warp-speed-vast-military-involvement. Accessed September 12, 2022.
8. LaFraniere S. Trump health aide pushes bizarre conspiracies and warns of armed revolt. *New York Times*. September 14, 2020. Available at: https://www.nytimes.com/2020/09/14/us/politics/caputo-virus.html. Accessed September 12, 2022.

9. Martin D. Operation Warp Speed: planning the distribution of a future COVID-19 vaccine. *60 Minutes*. November 9, 2020. Available at: https://www.youtube.com/watch?v= 240DMmhgp4M. Accessed September 12, 2022.

10. The Forum at Harvard T.H. Chan School of Public Health. Nancy Messonnier. January 11, 2021. Available at: https://theforum.sph.harvard.edu/expert-participants/nancy-messonnier. Accessed September 12, 2022.

11. Centers for Disease Control and Prevention. Transcript for the CDC telebriefing update on COVID-19. [Press briefing transcript]. February 26, 2020. Available at: https://www.cdc.gov/media/releases/2020/t0225-cdc-telebriefing-covid-19.html. Accessed September 12, 2022.

12 Werner E, Abutaleb Y, Sun LH, Bernstein L. Coronavirus's spread in US is "inevitable," CDC warns. *Washington Post*. February 28, 2020. Available at: https://www.washingtonpost.com/us-policy/2020/02/25/cdc-coronavirus-inevitable. Accessed September 12, 2022.

13. Moreno JE. Trump threatened to fire CDC's chief of respiratory diseases in February: report. *Hill*. April 22, 2020. Available at: https://thehill.com/homenews/administration/494187-trump-threatened-to-fire-cdcs-chief-of-respiratory-diseases-in. Accessed September 12, 2022.

14. US Government Accountability Office. COVID-19 HHS and DOD transitioned vaccine responsibilities to HHS, but need to address outstanding issues. January 2022. Available at: https://www.gao.gov/assets/gao-22-104453.pdf. Accessed September 24, 2022.

15. McKesson. McKesson to distribute future COVID-19 vaccines in support of Operation Warp Speed. August 14, 2020. Available at: https://www.mckesson.com/About-McKesson/Newsroom/Press-Releases/2020/McKesson-Distribute-Future-COVID-19-Vaccines-Operation-Warp-Speed/#:~:text=The-CDC-has-an-existing,the-event-of-a-pandemic. Accessed September 12, 2022.

16. Centers for Disease Control and Prevention. Crisis & Emergency Risk Communication (CERC). January 23, 2018. Available at: https://emergency.cdc.gov/cerc. Accessed September 12, 2022.

17. Diamond D. Messonnier, Birx detail political interference in last year's coronavirus response. *Washington Post*. November 12, 2021. Available at: https://www.washingtonpost.com/health/2021/11/12/messonnier-birx-coronavirus-response-interference. Accessed September 12, 2022.

18. House investigators release interview excerpts with Messonnier, Birx and others. *Washington Post*. Updated November 12, 2021. Available at: https://www.washingtonpost.com/context/house-investigators-release-interview-excerpts-with-messonnier-birx-and-others/d4efe499-329f-41c7-a3aa-0e06b0e52b94/?itid=lk_inline_manual_3. Accessed September 12, 2022.

19. Centers for Disease Control and Prevention. COVID-19 vaccination program interim playbook for jurisdiction operations. Version 1.0, September 16, 2020. Available at: https://stacks.cdc.gov/view/cdc/93806. Accessed September 12, 2022.

20. Stanley-Becker I, Sun LH. Senior CDC official who met Trump's wrath for raising alarm about coronavirus to resign. *Washington Post*. May 7, 2021. Available at: https://www.washingtonpost.com/health/2021/05/07/cdc-official-resigns. Accessed September 12, 2022.

21. US Department of State. White House Operation Warp Speed Vaccine Summit. December 8, 2020. Available at: https://www.youtube.com/watch?v=0yclESPhfIU. Accessed September 12, 2022.

22. Orenstein W. Vaccines don't save lives. Vaccinations save lives. *Hum Vaccin Immunother*. 2019;15(12):2786–2789. doi:10.1080/21645515.2019.1682360.

23. Banco E, Cancryn A. Top CDC official resigns from post following reassignment. *Politico*. Updated May 7, 2021. Available at: https://www.politico.com/news/2021/05/07/nancy-messonnier-resigns-485684. Accessed September 12, 2022.

24. Messonnier N. COVID-19 vaccine implementation. [PowerPoint]. Centers for Disease Control and Prevention. August 18, 2020. Available at: https://web.csg.org/tcs/wp-content/uploads/sites/13/2020/08/8.18.20-CDC-Implementation-Slides.pdf. Accessed September 12, 2022.

25. US Department of Health and Human Services. From the factory to the frontlines: the Operation Warp Speed strategy for distributing a COVID-19 vaccine. Available at: https://www.hhs.gov/sites/default/files/strategy-for-distributing-covid-19-vaccine.pdf. Accessed September 12, 2022.

26. Roussel A. Business as usual: Paul Mango of Operation Warp Speed. [Transcript]. Pittsburgh Technology Council. December 21, 2020. Available at: https://www.pghtech.org/programs/BAUxPaulMangoOpWarpSpeed. Accessed September 12, 2022.

27. C-SPAN. Paul Mango on the One-Year Anniversary of Operation Warp Speed. *Washington Journal*. December 17, 2021. Available at: https://www.c-span.org/video/?516748-5%2Fwashington-journal-paul-mango-discusses-year-anniversary-operation-warp-speed. Accessed September 12, 2022.

28. Centers for Disease Control and Prevention. Administration announces $200 million from CDC to jurisdictions for COVID-19 vaccine preparedness. [Press release]. September 23, 2020. Available at: https://www.cdc.gov/media/releases/2020/p0924-200-million-jurisdictions-covid-19-preparedness.html. Accessed September 12, 2022.

29. US Government Accountability Office. Influenza pandemic: lessons from the H1N1 pandemic should be incorporated into future planning. June 2011. Available at: https://www.gao.gov/assets/gao-11-632.pdf. Accessed September 23, 2022.

30. Association of Immunization Managers. Statement on the need for federal COVID-19 vaccine resources. September 9, 2020. Available at: https://www.immunizationmanagers.org/resources/statement-on-the-need-for-federal-covid-19-vaccine-resources. Accessed September 12, 2022.

31. Association of Immunization Managers. Immunization program leaders call for federal investment in COVID-19 vaccine distribution preparation. April 9, 2020. Available at: https://www.immunizationmanagers.org/resources/immunization-program-leaders-call-for-federal-investment-in-covid-19-vaccine-distribution-preparation. Accessed September 12, 2022.

32. US Congress, House Committee on Appropriations. H.R. 6074, Coronavirus Preparedness and Response Supplemental Appropriations Act, 2020: title-by-title summary. March 3, 2020. Available at: https://www.congress.gov/bill/116th-congress/house-bill/6074. Accessed October 7, 2022.

33. Congressional Research Service. US Public Health Service: COVID-19 supplemental appropriations in the 116th Congress. Updated August 3, 2021. Available at: https://sgp.fas.org/crs/misc/R46711.pdf. Accessed September 23, 2022.

34. Murray P. The Democratic COVID-19 response: a roadmap to getting a safe and effective vaccine to all. US Senate Committee on Health, Education, Labor, and Pensions. July 13, 2020. Available at: https://www.help.senate.gov/imo/media/doc/Murray-Vaccines-White-Paper-FINAL.pdf. Accessed September 12, 2022.

35. Spiro T, Emanuel Z. A comprehensive COVID-19 vaccine plan: efficient manufacturing, financing, and distribution of a COVID-19 vaccine. Center for American Progress. July 28, 2020. Available at: https://www.americanprogress.org/article/comprehensive-covid-19-vaccine-plan. Accessed September 12, 2022.

36. Rev. CDC director Robert Redfield coronavirus response Senate hearing transcript, September 16. September 16, 2020. Available at: https://www.rev.com/blog/transcripts/cdc-coronavirus-response-senate-hearing-transcript-september-16. Accessed September 12, 2022.

37. Sun LH. Top health official says states need about $6 billion from Congress to distribute coronavirus vaccine. *Washington Post*. September 16, 2020. Available at: https://www.washingtonpost.com/health/2020/09/16/vaccine-distribution-roadmap. Accessed September 12, 2022.

38. Florko N. Trump officials actively lobbied to deny states money for vaccine rollout last fall. *STAT*. January 31, 2021. Available at: https://www.statnews.com/2021/01/31/trump-officials-lobbied-to-deny-states-money-for-vaccine-rollout. Accessed September 12, 2022.

39. Centers for Disease Control and Prevention. COVID-19 vaccination planning: August letter to health departments, August 2, 2020.

40. Association of State and Territorial Health Officials and Association of Immunization Managers. Consideration of state and territorial "draw down" of COVID-19 vaccination funding memo to RADM Jerome Adams and senior HHS officials. December 4, 2020.

41. National Archives and Records Service. Public papers of the presidents of the United States, Dwight D. Eisenhower, 1957, containing the public messages, speeches, and statements of the president, remarks at the National Defense Executive Reserve Conference. November 14, 1957. Washington, DC: Federal Register Division, General Services Administration.

42. Quote Investigator. Plans are worthless, but planning is everything. Updated October 28, 2021. Available at: https://quoteinvestigator.com/2017/11/18/planning. Accessed September 12, 2022.

43. Consolidated Appropriations Act of 2021, HR 133, 116th Cong, (2020). Available at: https://www.congress.gov/116/plaws/publ260/PLAW-116publ260.pdf. Accessed September 12, 2022.

44. College of Physicians of Philadelphia. How are vaccines made? Vaccines for pandemic threats. Available at: https://historyofvaccines.org/vaccines-101/how-are-vaccines-made/vaccines-pandemic-threats. Accessed September 12, 2022.

45. Centers for Disease Control and Prevention, National Center for Immunization and Respiratory Diseases. Pandemic vaccine program: distribution, tracking, administration, and monitoring. 2020. Available at: https://www.cdc.gov/flu/pdf/pandemic-resources/pandemic-influenza-vaccine-distribution-9p-508.pdf. Accessed September 12, 2022.

46. Galen Institute. The inside story behind Operation Warp Speed. February 22, 2022. Available at: https://galen.org/2022/the-inside-story-behind-operation-warp-speed. Accessed September 12, 2022.

47. Lyons G. Tom Cotton wouldn't be anywhere without government dollars. *Arkansas Times*. October 9, 2014. Available at: https://arktimes.com/columns/gene-lyons/2014/10/09/tom-cotton-wouldnt-be-anywhere-without-government-dollars?oid=3479339. Accessed September 12, 2022.

5

Attending to a Thousand Details

So I imagine the beginning of this is going to be pretty chaotic. And I imagine a lot of places are going to be expecting a certain amount of vaccine and they're going to get a lot less. That's going to be frustrating for all the planners and it's going to be really frustrating for people who really want that vaccine early.[1]

–Former Assistant Secretary for Preparedness and
Response Dr. Nicole Lurie on COVID vaccine rollout

Exploding head emoji.[2]

–Text response from Claire Hannan to an immunization manager's question, "How are
we going to do this?" referring to cold storage requirements for new vaccines

On September 16, 2020, over four months after the launch of Operation Warp Speed (OWS), the Centers for Disease Control and Prevention (CDC) was finally cleared to release the *COVID-19 Vaccination Program Jurisdiction Operations Interim Operational Guidance*, known in short as the *CDC Playbook*. While criticized in some quarters for not including every detail in the vaccine distribution and administration process, and especially for its lack of inclusion of any budget to execute the plans, its release was a major turning point and accelerator in state and jurisdictional planning. The *CDC Playbook* also prompted consideration of a thousand details each jurisdiction would need to address in finalizing plans for local vaccine distribution.

Unlike earlier OWS updates, the playbook strongly reflected the CDC's perspective. It assured state and local public health officials that despite the months of apparent tension and debate between the CDC and OWS leaders, the national COVID distribution plan would largely build upon the existing vaccine distribution system. Under this scheme, publicly funded vaccines are delivered largely but not exclusively through private-sector partners.

After months of increasing frustration as states were trying to plan without much actionable information, the jurisdictions now found themselves in a scramble. The Department of Health and Human Services (HHS) announced that vaccines could be available as early as November, and accordingly the *CDC Playbook* included a requirement for jurisdictions to draft and submit a plan in response to the new guidance within 30 days.

The CDC's guidance included a carefully worded overview of the COVID vaccination program's ultimate goals. Vaccination was part of the US strategy to "reduce COVID-19-related illnesses, hospitalizations, and deaths and to help restore societal functioning.

The goal of the US government is to have enough COVID-19 vaccine for all people in the United States who wish to be vaccinated."[3(p5)] It also set out to manage expectations, stating, "Early in the COVID-19 vaccination program, there may be a limited supply of COVID-19 vaccine, and vaccination efforts may focus on those critical to the response, providing direct care, and maintaining societal function, as well as those at highest risk for developing severe illness from COVID-19."[3(p5)] Notably, it did not set a goal of achieving herd immunity.

Over 15 sections and 75 pages in length, the *CDC Playbook* covered all aspects of public health preparedness planning, including standing up an organizational structure and assuring partner involvement, anticipating a planned phased approach to COVID-19 vaccination, and acknowledging the need to identify and prioritize critical populations. It included recommendations for COVID-19 vaccination provider recruitment and enrollment, understanding a jurisdiction's COVID-19 vaccine administration capacity, and what to expect regarding COVID-19 vaccine allocation, ordering, distribution, and inventory management. The guidance also highlighted the extraordinary COVID-19 vaccine storage and handling requirement and the critical vaccine administration documentation and reporting procedures. As well, it included plans for vaccination second-dose reminders and requirements for immunization information systems and other external data systems. Finally, it included an overview of vaccination program communications, regulatory and safety considerations, and vaccine program monitoring.

Notably, the *CDC Playbook* did not include projections of vaccine supply, targets of how many Americans might be vaccinated by any future date, or specific details on who would be prioritized to receive the vaccine first; and perhaps most important, it included no indication of what resources would be available to implement the plans states and jurisdictions were being asked to develop within 30 days of its release. Along with the *CDC Playbook*, HHS also released the OWS companion document entitled *From the Factory to the Frontlines*.[4] This document, described as a report to Congress to detail a strategy for delivering the COVID vaccine to every American who wants it, summarized much of what was included in the *CDC Playbook*.

One of the most welcome announcements included in both strategy documents was the official confirmation that the plan was to largely utilize the existing vaccine delivery infrastructure, the system that CDC and state and local jurisdictions had been urging from the start. The *Factory to Frontlines* plan stated:

> OWS is harnessing the strength of existing vaccine delivery infrastructure while leveraging innovative strategies, new public-private partnerships, and robust engagement of state, local, tribal, and territorial health departments to ensure efficient, effective, and equitable access to COVID-19 vaccines.[4(p1)]

Jurisdictions finally had the reassurance that they would not have to reinvent existing vaccine delivery systems, although the immensity of work to operationalize the plans called for in the *CDC Playbook* became quickly apparent.

A NATIONAL STRATEGY EMERGES

In a brief 11 pages, the *Factory to Frontlines* strategy spelled out a vision for how the national vaccine distribution campaign would unfold. According to the plan, four key tasks were necessary to achieving the primary objective of ensuring vaccine access for every American who wants it:

1. Continue engaging with state, tribal, territorial, and local partners, other stakeholders, and the public to communicate public health information, before and after distribution begins, around the vaccine and promote vaccine confidence and uptake.
2. Distribute vaccines immediately upon granting of Emergency Use Authorization/Biologics License Application, using a transparently developed, phased allocation methodology.
3. Ensure safe administration of the vaccine and availability of administration supplies.
4. Monitor necessary data from the vaccination program through an information technology (IT) system capable of supporting and tracking distribution, administration, and other necessary data.[4(p2)]

The document recounted how a federal team had worked with five pilot jurisdictions—California, Florida, Minnesota, North Dakota, and Philadelphia—to "utilize a basic plan for administration and adapt it to create jurisdiction-specific plans that will serve as models for other jurisdictions."[4(p3)] It indicated how jurisdictional planning would cover coordination with federal facilities in their jurisdiction, coordination with national chain partners, vaccination of critical workforces, and ways to reach underserved populations. It also highlighted how each jurisdiction would be required to develop a "micro plan" based on their existing plans as well as outputs from the first five jurisdictions supported, with CDC providing technical assistance. These micro plans were to identify vaccination sites and necessary logistical considerations and lay out how the sites would be onboarded into the necessary information technology system.

The strategy also highlighted how centralized distribution would allow "the government full visibility, control, and ability to shift assets and use data to optimize vaccine uptake."[4(p4)] Noting that McKesson had also served as the centralized distributor for the H1N1 vaccine in 2009, the plan confirmed that once vaccines were allocated to a given jurisdiction or authorized partner, McKesson would deliver a specific amount of vaccine to a designated location. In many instances, delivery locations were the sites where the vaccine would be administered, but the plan provided that vaccines could also be delivered to locations in jurisdictions to be further distributed to administration sites within health department networks.

As for delivery sites, the document noted, "Successful delivery of this vaccine will need to incorporate new types of sites and approaches for vaccine delivery."[4(p4)] It highlighted the expected major role for pharmacies, saying, "During H1N1, once vaccines became widely available pharmacies played an important role in the vaccine distribution; pharmacies' role is even more critical to vaccinations today and will be fully integrated into the distribution plan."[4(p4)] Dr. Mitchel Rothholz, chief of governance and state affiliates at the American Pharmacists Association (APhA), shared additional background on the evolution of pharmacists' role in vaccination. "We set up a guiding principle that we weren't coming in to disrupt but to complement. We actually created the concept of the immunization neighborhood, and I think that has been embraced by public health and others" (author oral interview with Mitchel Rothholz, RPh, MBA, February 25, 2022).

But because for COVID so many pharmacies were new to the system and having a venue for coordination was lacking, both Rothholz (APhA) and Blumenstock (ASTHO) were instrumental in forming a collaboration of health care and public health organizations called the National Associations' COVID Vaccine Leadership Council to support implementation of the nation's COVID-19 vaccination plan. The council created a forum to strategize, discuss, exchange, and work toward solving some of the challenges expected as jurisdictions implemented the CDC's COVID-19 vaccination playbook at the state level. Upon the launch, Blumenstock said:

> This is a monumental task. We must make sure that we're collaborating across traditional public health and healthcare sectors so that we're ready to effectively and efficiently distribute and administer the approved vaccines. Our united approach will make the process more effective and efficient, our nation stronger, and communities safer. We want to give the public confidence and enhance public trust in the vaccination process.[5]

The COVID Vaccine Leadership Council would prove to be an effective forum for problem solving throughout the campaign in coordination of efforts between state and local government agencies, the pharmacy sector, and health care providers and health insurers.

The scope and scale of the vaccine distribution and administration process was mind boggling. State and local health officials and their health care and pharmacy partners had to consider thousands of details as they readied their jurisdictions and organizations for the vaccine campaign. While plans had finally been shared, many uncertainties and unknowns remained that still meant contingency plans were needed. These details presented themselves in many areas, including ordering and tracking; phased implementation; allocation and prioritization; vaccine administration, monitoring, and engagement; communication; and confidence.

ORDERING AND TRACKING

The *Factory to Frontlines* strategy also provided an overview of the nuts and bolts of how the vaccine would get from the point of manufacturing to its administration by local providers in medical care, public health clinics, and pharmacies. It confirmed that vaccine allocation and centralized distribution would utilize CDC's existing vaccine tracking system, called VTrckS, which is a secure, web-based IT system that integrates the entire publicly funded vaccine supply chain from purchasing and ordering through distribution to participating state, local, and territorial health departments and to health care providers. VTrckS would be scaled for the distribution of pandemic vaccines, to include the onboarding of new providers under each jurisdiction's micro plan.

For the COVID-19 vaccination program, additional providers, including private partners (e.g., pharmacy chains) and other federal entities (e.g., the HHS Indian Health Service), would be onboarded to enable allocation to and ordering directly by these partners, in addition to the state, local, and territorial allocations. Through the linkage of several systems, information technology was also envisioned to help direct people to where to get vaccinated using a web-based "finder" system.

PHASED IMPLEMENTATION

The strategy anticipated that vaccine rollout would proceed over three phases. Phase 1 would begin upon Food and Drug Administration (FDA) authorization when "initial vaccine doses would be distributed in a focused manner, with the goal of maximizing vaccine acceptance and public health protection while minimizing waste and inefficiency."[4(p5)] It was anticipated that this phase would be marked by a highly constrained supply that would require vaccines to be administered mostly in closed settings such as hospitals and other worksite-based settings. States were told this phase could begin as early as November 2020. While this created some anxiety in terms of the need for quick preparation, the concept of planning for phases created some relief that jurisdictions could continue planning for Phase 2 while Phase 1 was underway. This scheme also allowed jurisdictions to prioritize which providers they needed to enroll and onboard first.

The strategy then envisioned that Phase 2 would begin as the volume of available vaccines increased and distribution would expand, increasing access to the larger population. The plan stated, "When larger quantities of vaccine become available, there will be two simultaneous objectives: (1) to provide widespread access to vaccination and achieve coverage across the US population and (2) to ensure high uptake in target populations, particularly those who are at high risk for severe outcomes from COVID-19."[4(p5)] It was anticipated that during this phase vaccine supply would rapidly increase and then exceed demand. Increased supply would allow jurisdictions to expand eligibility beyond the initial prioritized populations and would allow a vaccine to be administered through commercial and private-sector partners (e.g., pharmacies, doctors' offices, clinics) as well as through public health sites, including mobile clinics, Federally Qualified Health Centers, and targeted community sites as needed.

For Phase 3, the plan anticipated that "if the risk of COVID-19 persists such that there remains a public health need for an ongoing vaccination program, COVID-19 vaccines will ultimately be universally available and integrated into routine vaccination programs, run by both public and private partners."[4(p5)] In this phase, there would be an excess supply of vaccines, thereby allowing broad immunization provider networks, no limits on eligibility, and likely little need for mass clinics.

ALLOCATION AND PRIORITIZATION

To support the prioritization of populations envisioned in the three phases, the federal strategy described the expected role of the CDC's Advisory Committee on Immunization Practice (ACIP). The plan stated that "ACIP will review evidence on COVID-19 epidemiology and burden, vaccine safety, vaccine efficacy, evidence quality, and implementation issues to inform recommendations for COVID-19 vaccine policy, including priority groups for vaccination, which are submitted to the CDC director for adoption."[4(p6)] This provided a critical clarification of the delicate and ethically fraught process to determine who should be first in line to receive a lifesaving vaccine when supply would be extremely limited. It also meant that priority groups would be set nationally as opposed to state by state.

The discussion noted that CDC was applying lessons learned from the H1N1 flu vaccine allocation program, which had been marked by manufacturing delays. The main lesson, CDC stated presciently, was that public health agencies need to anticipate delays and respond to changing circumstances. Despite the OWS leadership's earlier dismissal of CDC's advocacy to include funding for "unforeseen circumstances," the strategy now acknowledged that "nimble delivery and allocation strategies will be essential."[4(p6)]

States have a long-standing familiarity with ACIP's critical role in providing gold-standard recommendations on the prioritization and use of all vaccines, including during the 2009 H1N1 pandemic. However, a curious incident happened earlier in July 2020 that, while perhaps well intentioned, demonstrated the drawbacks of having too many cooks in the proverbial kitchen. In mid-July, Dr. Francis Collins, the widely esteemed director of the National Institutes of Health (NIH), announced that he was requesting the prestigious National Academy of Medicine (NAM) to convene an expert panel to develop a framework to determine who should be vaccinated first.[6] The problem was that this task directly overlapped with the charge to the CDC's ACIP. The NIH's overlap with ACIP's work, combined with murky statements from OWS leaders about their potential role in determining allocation priorities, created confusion and heightened anxiety among public health officials. "It seems to me like we've just assigned four different air traffic control towers to land the same plane,"[6] Dr. Michael Osterholm, director of the University of Minnesota's Center for Infectious Diseases Research and Policy, told *STAT News* that July. In that same story, Dr. Collins indicated that he was motivated to create an advisory process outside of government to build trust.

The statement by Dr. Collins is not surprising given his credentials in science, but it overlooks that the CDC's ACIP is explicitly constituted as an independent advisory body of experts for this same purpose. In addition to the 15 voting members, ACIP includes 8 nonvoting ex officio members who represent other federal agencies with responsibility for immunization programs in the United States. Also included are 30 nonvoting representatives of liaison organizations that bring related immunization expertise and assure that the perspective of those who will implement the ACIP recommendations are included in their predecisional deliberations. While it would be possible for NAM to recreate all these important linkages, the fact that it was being asked to do so by a representative of the federal government involved in OWS reinforced significant concerns among state and local officials about a lack of coordination and potential for duplication.

As the NAM process unfolded, the academy appointed Drs. Bill Foege and Helene Gayle, a former CDC director and a CDC AIDS Division director, respectively, as cochairs. This defused some of the concern about the group because of their intimate knowledge of the CDC and ACIP relationship. Over several months, the NAM study group deliberated and produced a solid set of recommendations,[7] with an admirable in-depth focus on achieving equity, although how much the ACIP relied on NAM's work is not apparent.

VACCINE ADMINISTRATION

The heart of the strategy was contained in the section on vaccine administration. As noted previously, vaccines do not save lives, vaccinations do. Therefore, all the work to develop, manufacture, and deliver safe and effective vaccines hinged on the part of the strategy focused on administering vaccine into the arms of willing Americans. The strategy outlined four key elements:

- Delivery of vaccine to sites, with the goal of no upfront costs to providers and no out-of-pocket cost to the vaccine recipient.
- Ensuring administration sites, as covered in the jurisdiction's micro plans, have the capabilities for storing, handling, and administering vaccine products with specific distribution and administration requirements.
- Supporting reliable distribution of ancillary supplies that may be necessary for vaccine administration.
- Engagement of traditional and nontraditional administration sites and approaches in vaccination planning to allow for flexibility to accommodate vaccine requirements.[4(p7)]

There is ample evidence that financial barriers to vaccines make it much more difficult for individuals to receive all recommended immunizations. Therefore, when this strategy was released in September 2020, many public health professionals welcomed the announcement that vaccine distribution would not entail any upfront costs for either providers or consumers. At the same time, the lack of details about financial reimbursement levels and mechanisms for a vaccine that was expected within months was another key missing component that created anxiety among state and local program officials.

Although not widely debated at the time, the characterization of the vaccine as being free obscured the fact that the vaccine was indeed being financed in full by US taxpayers. This raises intriguing questions about how people value public health services that we all necessarily pay for out of taxes rather than individually out of pocket. Would more individuals have been vaccinated if the vaccines were assigned their real value or if consumers were told how much each vaccine and its administration cost?

Equally important to assuring no out-of-pocket costs to consumers, the strategy spelled out a commitment to making access to vaccines as convenient as possible. It detailed how Phase 1 vaccinations would largely take place in closed clinics that would be targeted exclusively for a class of prioritized workers or individuals, such as hospitals, health systems, or places of employment for essential workers. Then, as Phase 2 progressed and vaccine supply rapidly increased, the strategy called for states and jurisdictions to recruit and enroll broad networks of community-based providers. These ranged from hospitals, doctors' offices, and mobile clinics to mass vaccination sites, all of which would receive vaccines from the state's allocation. This network would be supplemented by capacity in pharmacies, long-term care and home health providers, the Indian Health Service, and other federal entities that would receive vaccines through a direct federal allocation. Jurisdictions welcomed this focus on building an extensive network of providers to reach all communities and immediately understood that close coordination would be necessary to provide maximum visibility as to where vaccines would be available in each community.

DATA AND MONITORING

To provide this visibility, the *Factory to Frontlines* plan stressed the importance of enhancing an information technology ecosystem to allow all stakeholders to monitor vaccine distribution. The strategy stated:

> The vaccination program requires extensive data monitoring infrastructure, including appropriate IT architecture, to incorporate claims and payment processes, to identify when a person needs a potential second dose, to monitor outcomes and adverse events, and to account for products the US government is spending billions of dollars to research, develop, and produce . . . Data will need to be available both federally and at the state, local, and tribal level to ensure efficient management of the vaccination program . . . OWS will construct and integrate an IT architecture that achieves this objective, building off of existing IT infrastructure and filling gaps with new IT solutions.[4(p9)]

From the outset, building a workable information technology infrastructure to support COVID vaccine distribution was one of the jurisdiction's biggest challenges. It ultimately turned out to be one of the biggest keys to success and necessitated much heavy lifting and technical wizardry to link together a system to reliably monitor the distribution and administration of hundreds of millions of vaccine doses.

The *Factory to Frontlines* strategy noted that the immunization information systems (IIS) used by state, territorial, and city entities that deliver public vaccinations would be central to this IT infrastructure. But jurisdictions knew that while IIS were generally developed to monitor routine childhood vaccinations, there were many gaps when it came to adult immunization provider networks. While most doctors' offices utilize some sort of electronic health record and the pharmaceutical chains have similar systems for their patients, the ability to link all the systems together and to integrate them with vaccine ordering, delivery, and inventory management systems was highly variable. A Congressional Research Service analysis of the utilization of IIS in the COVID vaccine program noted that one priority was to ensure that providers that had not typically administered vaccine before the pandemic, including many pharmacies, long-term care facilities, and mass vaccination sites, were quickly trained to do so.[8]

Additional controversy occurred when, in late 2020, the CDC asked states to submit personally identifiable information on vaccine recipients to CDC's data clearinghouse. Several states objected, causing CDC to create several agreements specific to each jurisdiction's concerns. Many state laws prohibit the sharing of personally identifiable information, and jurisdictions are extremely careful about following their data-sharing policies, and so typically states report de-identified information to federal health authorities. The incident underscored the highly sensitive subject of what personally identifiable health information the government collects; how that information is protected, shared, and utilized; and fears about the creation of anything resembling a national database. Without the flexibility shown by CDC to address jurisdictions' concerns, the controversy could have exacerbated the already considerable misinformation and accompanying hesitation.

In addition, OWS introduced a new data system called Tiberius just weeks before the vaccine launch. This system was intended to provide end-to-end visibility of all vaccine doses throughout the distribution and administration process. Many found the system to provide useful insights. However, most states surveyed by *USA Today* said the data Tiberius provides on demographics and vulnerable populations "is less detailed than data they already have on hand. Some also criticized the timing, saying the system came too late and was too complex to learn in time for the vaccine rollout."[9] The *USA Today* review concluded that "many of the health officials who make the final decisions on who gets the vaccine, at the county, city and other local levels, aren't using the system at all."[9] Anticipating these challenges, the *Factory to Frontlines* strategy signaled that this would be an area in need of great attention.

ENGAGEMENT, COMMUNICATION, AND CONFIDENCE

The *Factory to Frontlines* strategy concluded with a section declaring the government's intentions regarding public engagement, communications, and promotion of vaccine confidence, stating:

> Working with established partners—especially those that are trusted sources for target audiences—is critical to advancing public understanding of, access to, and acceptance of eventual vaccines . . . To build partnerships as part of the vaccination program and deliver an effective communications strategy, OWS is engaging public, nonprofit, and private partners, while leveraging the government's longstanding relationships with state health departments, tribal nations and organizations, healthcare systems, the vaccine industry, health insurance issuers and plans, and non-traditional partners.[4(p10)]

While the focus was on target, the reference to leveraging long-standing relationships with state health departments rang a bit hollow, considering how states had been excluded from the early OWS planning process. Nevertheless, the strategy finally gave long-overdue acknowledgment of the CDC's track record in safely distributing vaccines to approximately 40,000 public and private providers across the country in addition to tens of millions of vaccines distributed through other channels. It referenced how CDC had expanded this capacity to 70,000 provider sites during the 2009 flu pandemic and said, "This represents strong baseline capacity and partnerships for distribution and administration."[4(p10)]

The final two sections of *Factory to Frontlines* stressed the importance of a strategic communications campaign and a concerted effort to promote vaccine confidence. For communications, the document stated that an information campaign would be run by the HHS Public Affairs Office rather than CDC (the leader of which, Michael Caputo, was mentioned in the last chapter for his belief that CDC scientists wearing sweatpants were plotting against Trump[10]). This assignment, though little noticed at the time, reflected the CDC's inability once again to convince OWS leaders that CDC had the capacity and expertise to conduct the critical communications campaign. The CDC had since May presented a proposed communications plan to the OWS leadership but apparently never received approval to proceed.

At first, the go-ahead for CDC to implement was not granted because of Dr. Slaoui's purported position that nothing should be communicated to the public until more details of the successful vaccine candidates were known. While some critical details, particularly for storage, handling, and number and timing of doses, would depend on the specific characteristics of a vaccine, so many areas of communications and planning were necessary regardless of the final vaccines approved. His apparent veto of the CDC communications plan was another key cause of overall planning delays and ultimate readiness. Nevertheless, the strategy noted the focus of the campaign would be on promoting vaccine safety and efficacy and targeting key populations and communities to ensure maximum vaccine acceptance.

Finally, regarding vaccine confidence, the strategy referenced the opportunity to utilize the CDC's existing Vaccinate with Confidence framework. It stressed the three key priorities: protect communities, empower families, and stop myths. The entire strategy closed by noting that the CDC was already working with local partners and using trusted messengers to establish new partnerships and contain the spread of misinformation. This was a battle that was about to intensify significantly.

THIRTY DAYS FOR JURISDICTIONAL PLANS

While not comprehensive, the combination of the *Factory to Frontlines* strategy and *CDC Playbook* provided jurisdictions with new details and a framework to expand their nascent planning assumptions. After waiting months for such guidance, states were given just 30 days to write and submit to CDC a plan in response. Plans would be reviewed by federal staff and summaries of each posted on the CDC website.[11] The CDC directed all 64 funded jurisdictions to "address all requirements outlined in the playbook and clearly describe their responsibility for ensuring activities are implemented."[3(p5)] The rush to require plans to be submitted three weeks before the 2020 presidential election also heightened concern in some quarters that the Trump administration would exert political influence on the FDA to approve a vaccine before all clinical trial safety data could be fully considered, so states had to demonstrate they were prepared.

While the guidance provided many long-awaited details, it also acknowledged that there were still many unknowns and uncertainties. These included a lack of information on any developmental vaccine's timing, quantity, and efficacy. Indeed, the guidance was designated "interim," with the promise of additional information when available. These unknown factors crystallized the immense challenges in providing a new vaccine to every American amid a global pandemic.

As states and jurisdictions drafted their plans in response to the *CDC Playbook*, they quickly recognized that the scale and scope of COVID created at least three major new challenges compared to H1N1. First, most new providers enrolled in the 2009 H1N1 pandemic effort had not maintained formal ties or had not remained registered with state immunization programs. Second, few states had conducted full-scale exercises involving all the vaccinators that would be needed for such a massive vaccination effort. Third, while 80 million doses of the H1N1 influenza vaccine were successfully distributed in 2009, the estimated number of doses needed to vaccinate the entire 2021 population of the United States exceeded 600 million. Immunization program managers realized early that the scale of planning for COVID would need to go well beyond any previous immunization campaign.

Despite these uncertainties and unprecedented challenges, many state and local immunization program leaders across the jurisdictions felt a sense of exhilaration that finally they could begin a detailed planning process. They felt as if their life's work building immunization programs would soon be in the national and even global spotlight. They knew that lives were at stake and that failure would not be an option. Michele Roberts typified the can-do spirit that infused the frantic planning in late 2020, saying, "We know how to do this. We will be ready" (author oral interview with Michele Roberts, MPH, MSHES, December 28, 2021).

THE FINAL BUILDUP

All jurisdictions submitted plans to CDC by the October 16 deadline. The CDC led an interagency review of these plans and synthesized some top strengths and challenges, which were presented to an ACIP meeting on October 30, 2020. Identified strengths included jurisdictions' embrace of the phased approach to vaccine rollout, the CDC's clear plans to train and equip providers to utilize the Vaccine Adverse Events Reporting System (VAERS) to support safety monitoring, and the provision of "deep operational detail" in support of second-dose reminder systems.[12] The three leading challenges identified at that time were a lack of detailed plans for communicating about the vaccine, the need to assure that all data systems were in place to support program monitoring, and the ability to enroll adequate provider networks to assure equitable vaccine access in later phases.

Then, at just about the same time the *CDC Playbook* jurisdiction plans were due, AIM conducted a webinar with representatives of Pfizer. On that webinar, company representatives for the first time shared details about the extraordinarily complex storage and handling requirements for their developmental vaccine. Pfizer explained that their vaccine needs to be stored at about −75°C, which is about 50 degrees colder than required for any vaccine currently used in the United States. Jurisdictions learned that once sites receive their thermal shippers filled with vials of vaccine, they are required to replenish the dry ice within 24 hours. If they do not use the vaccine within five days, they need to replenish the dry ice again, and once again five days later. The jurisdictions were informed that sites can use the shipper to store the vaccine until doses are ready to thaw, dilute, and inject into arms. This information simultaneously stoked concerns about dry ice availability and shortages while calming fears about the need to acquire ultracold freezers.

Jurisdictions also learned that the process requires vaccinators to act fast when removing vaccine from the shippers because, according to Pfizer's instructions, the boxes may be opened only twice a day, and each time for no more than a minute to ensure a constant temperature. At any point, the vaccine can be removed from the shipper and put in the refrigerator, but the vaccine can stay in the refrigerator for only up to five days before it expires. If not used within that window, the vaccines would have to be thrown away. According to the overview, when the vaccine is ready to use, nurses or other clinicians need to dilute it to make five doses per vial. Those five shots must be given within six hours. If more than six hours pass, the vaccines must be thrown out. And if that were not complex enough, the whole process must be repeated for each recipient, since the vaccine is given in two doses spaced three weeks apart.

To the immunization program officials listening, it became immediately apparent that this vaccine had extraordinary complex storage and handling requirements. In his book recounting Pfizer's role in COVID vaccine development, Pfizer CEO Dr. Albert Bourla said, "Manufacturing the vaccine had left us with a product as fragile as a snowflake. We now had to deliver that snowflake with great care around the world."[13(p93)] State and local jurisdictions were now being asked to deliver and administer tens of millions of these snowflakes. Claire Hannan recalls thinking then that the challenges her members would need to surmount to deliver COVID vaccine were unprecedented. In a story later picked up by CNN, she received a text inquiry from Molly Howell, the immunization program manager in North Dakota, asking, "How are we going to do this?" Hannan responded with an exploding head emoji.[2]

But after hearing that Pfizer had developed a special ultracold thermal shipping box with an extensive temperature and GPS monitoring system, a sense of optimism returned. At the end of the exploding head emoji story, Dr. Kelly Moore told CNN about the resourcefulness of her former colleagues. "It's going to be hard. Mistakes will be made, but we will learn from them, and we will get better and better," she said. Howell added, "It's a very big deal. I think we can do it."[2]

POLITICS, DELIVERY DATES, AND ACCELERATED TIMELINES

One of the most difficult elements that state and local jurisdictions faced in the planning process was uncertainty about when they would receive the first shipments of vaccine and how many doses to expect. When President Trump announced OWS in May 2020, he indicated that the projected timeline was "by the end of the year."[14] Regarding the amount of expected vaccine, Dr. Moncef Slaoui stated at the OWS launch, "I have very recently seen early data from a clinical trial with a coronavirus vaccine. And this data made me feel even more confident that we will be able to deliver a few hundred million doses of vaccine by the end of 2020."[14]

Throughout the summer, during an increasingly contentious campaign, the president raised the prospect that vaccines could be widely available before November 3, Election Day. This continued to ratchet up fears that the administration was willing to pressure and perhaps interfere with the FDA's rigorous scientific review and approval processes. At an Arizona tele-rally on July 18, 2020, the president declared, "We expect to have

100 million doses of vaccine available before the end of the year and maybe much sooner than that."[15]

A few weeks later, on August 4, the CDC issued a letter from Dr. Nancy Messonnier to immunization program jurisdictions conveying updated planning assumptions. The communication said that "limited COVID-19 vaccine doses will be available in fall 2020"[16] and that initial populations recommended for vaccination "would likely be those in the critical workforce who provide health care and maintain essential functions of society and staff and residents in long term care facilities."[16] Despite the CDC's efforts to set realistic expectations about limited vaccine availability at the outset of the vaccine rollout, the president once again ratcheted up the political pressure on the agency in his own government charged with assuring the safety of any vaccine. On Saturday, August 22, he sent a tweet that confirmed many fears that he was explicitly creating an artificial deadline for FDA action before the election:

> The deep state, or whoever, over at the FDA is making it very difficult for drug companies to get people in order to test the vaccines and therapeutics. Obviously, they are hoping to delay the answer until after November 3rd. Must focus on speed, and saving lives![17]

The pharmaceutical industry immediately pushed back with a strong defense of why the FDA needed to remain independent to maintain trust that no corners were being cut in the review and approval processes. Nevertheless, in September, President Trump echoed his July prediction in a White House press briefing, saying, "We'll have manufactured at least 100 million vaccine doses before the end of the year and likely much more than that. Hundreds of millions of doses will be available every month . . . And numbers that I'm telling you today, I think we'll exceed them very, very substantially."[18]

While the administration was offering optimistic estimates on the timing and amount of vaccine, the number of unanswered questions about distribution among state and local officials continued to multiply. Earlier in the year, OWS had set up regular but parallel communications channels with the jurisdictions to provide regular forums to provide planning updates and receive questions from those closest to the front lines. To their credit, OWS leaders recognized the critical importance of keeping governors and their staff involved and in the loop.

Carrying out the most important and logistically challenging public health operation in a century needed a high degree of executive leadership and political will to be successful, yet this was not being achieved. For example, CDC conducted at least weekly calls between CDC leaders and the immunization program staff. Rarely if ever were all the key stakeholders on the same call at the same time. This resulted in uneven situational awareness and sometimes conflicting and uncoordinated communication between federal and state partners.

One of the key factors OWS leaders did not seem to account for in engaging exclusively with governors is that the tactical and predecisional work of implementing public health policy and programs does not occur at the executive level. Instead, most state health officials and their programmatic staff are tasked with devising a health response strategy, advising and executing COVID policy decisions, as well as working directly with federal response partners at the CDC, FDA, HHS Office of the Assistant Secretary of Health, Centers for Medicare and Medicaid Services, Indian Health Service, and Health Resources and Services Administration, and in particular the regional staff of these entities. Communications directly to governors, but not directly with their health officials and health agency leadership, caused several notable instances in which immunization program staff were informed by their colleagues in their governor's office of a decision or policy update shared on an OWS call that either undermined or conflicted with information being shared on CDC calls.

Furthermore, despite the regular communications between OWS leaders and state governors, by the middle of October the states' frustration with the lack of clarity on many key planning elements boiled over. This caused the National Governors Association (NGA) to issue a press release and publicly post a list of pressing questions that still lacked answers despite the administration's drumbeat that tens of millions of doses of vaccine would be authorized and delivered shortly and their prior planning guidance shared with states. The NGA press release sharing the questions said governors and their teams were

seeking clarity on how to most effectively distribute and administer a COVID-19 vaccine. The distribution and implementation of the vaccine is a massive undertaking that cannot be managed without significant logistical coordination, planning and financial assistance between states and the federal government. The list of questions—which were submitted from Republican and Democratic governors from around the country—covers funding for the administration of a vaccine, allocation, and supply chain, and communication and information requirements.[19]

It was a troubling sign that even after the release of the *CDC Playbook* and the requirement for every jurisdiction to submit a plan, so many aspects of the vaccine rollout still appeared to be unsettled. The release continued:

The National Governors Association . . . sent a letter to the president of the United States last week. We asked to meet with the president to discuss how this is supposed to work between the federal government and the states. We are now releasing a compilation of questions from governors all across the country, Democratic and Republican, saying to the White House: how is this going to work? We need to answer these questions before the vaccine is available so that we are ready to go and no one is caught flat-footed when the time comes to vaccinate people.[19]

This episode was notable for reflecting what in Washington is known as negotiation by press release. This tactic is often resorted to when requested private conversations are either not taking place or are unsatisfactory. The hope is that public disclosure will focus attention and bring forth answers. The release's reference to making sure "no one is caught flat-footed"[19] is also a possible indication that governors were anticipating and perhaps trying to preempt the expected finger-pointing that often occurs when coordination between federal and state action is less than optimal.

While the list of outstanding questions from the NGA covered the range of vaccine distribution activities, it was also striking that the first seven questions all focused on the lack of funding provided to states up until that time. The questions reflected the huge divide between what the states judged their needs to be and the position OWS leaders took—namely, that since the vaccine and supplies were already paid for, the states did not need any additional money to coordinate distribution. The governors had a long list of top-priority funding questions, such as these:

- Will there be funding allocated to states to assist with distribution of the vaccine and other vaccine efforts?
- Without additional state and local funding to implement COVID-19 vaccine plans, we will be hampered in what we can accomplish. When can we expect more definitive information about resources related to this response?
- What are the plans for any federal contracts and/or additional funding to support "boots on the ground" to vaccinate in tier 2 and beyond?
- How will vaccine administration costs be covered for people who are uninsured?
- Will the federal government be setting guidelines around allowable vaccine administration costs for those with health insurance (whether that is state insurance, Medicaid, Medicare, CHIP, or some other state funded health insurance)?
- How will funding/reimbursement for vaccines be handled?
- We understand that the vaccine will initially be provided at no cost, as was remdesivir. However, states now must pay for remdesivir on the commercial market. How long will the federal government commit to providing the vaccine to states cost-free?[19]

In response, HHS publicly posted answers to each of the NGA questions online.[20] However, the response to the questions about funding for states reflected the wide gap in understanding between the federal and state partners. Citing the $340 million already allocated to the states, the HHS response essentially told states not to worry, writing:

In considering funding needs, states should recognize that most of the major costs of a vaccine campaign are already being covered. For example:

1. Securing vaccines and most accompanying supplies will cost the state nothing as these are paid for by the federal government;
2. Almost all transportation of a vaccine is covered, either through the manufacturer or through McKesson, the contractor being paid to move the vaccine to administration sites throughout the country;
3. Providers who administer the vaccine will be paid through insurance reimbursement under Medicare and Medicaid, or private coverage;

4. Healthcare providers who vaccinate uninsured persons will receive reimbursement through the federal uninsured fund managed by the Health Resources and Services Administration (HRSA), which has already been covering the cost of care for uninsured COVID-19 patients; and

5. Training for most of the healthcare provider workforce to administer the vaccine will be covered in large part by their employing institutions, be it hospitals, pharmacy chains, or other large healthcare entities.[20]

In other words, despite issuing a 75-page playbook spelling out 15 discrete areas that jurisdictions were charged with coordinating to assure a successful vaccination campaign, HHS was still trying to convince its state and local partners on the eve of the largest public health campaign in American history that they did not require any additional resources.

While it is impossible to know for certain if the rollout would have been smoother had the money for public health activities been provided earlier, the lack of resources provided to the front lines in the home stretch of the development process and leading up to vaccine distribution was clearly one of the biggest hurdles states faced in their planning.

Despite the lack of dedicated funding resources, the expectations placed on jurisdictions continued to mount. One week before the 2020 presidential election, the CDC issued another update for state and local public health agencies, saying, "In order to increase readiness at all levels, we ask that all jurisdictions plan to be ready to receive vaccine by November 15."[21] Although the letter gave the jurisdictions no indication of approximately how much vaccine to be ready to receive, it did lay out a prioritized list of five key planning updates to prepare "to implement this vaccination mission" (written communication with Claire Hannan, MPH, internal communication to Association of Immunization Managers, October 2020). No specific details were provided as to why the CDC set a November 15 date.

The first action to ensure readiness was for each jurisdiction to return a signed Data Use Agreement (DUA) for data sharing with CDC. The letter acknowledged that "the data architecture to support COVID-19 response is complex."[21] It stated that the response required at a minimum a DUA with CDC for reporting data to the COVID-19 Clearinghouse and Immunization Data Lake. This data sharing would be essential in tracking national uptake, identifying pockets of low vaccination, intervening in coverage disparities, and allocating vaccine supply. The second requested action was to enumerate the sites "prioritized to receive and administer vaccine A, a product that requires ultracold ($-60°C$ to $-80°C$) storage."[21] Noting that health care personnel would likely be among those prioritized for early vaccination, this request essentially asked states to canvas which and how many hospitals had storage capacity and referenced an earlier ultracold-temperature vaccine template that CDC had circulated to assess vaccine storage capacity.

The third priority request was for states to identify up to five priority locations for potentially prepositioning vaccines. This came in response to an OWS push to ensure that supply would be close to administration sites. Vaccines would be delivered and prepositioned before the FDA issued emergency use authorization and before the Advisory Committee on Immunization Practices issued its prioritization and use recommendations. The goal was to shorten the timeline between FDA authorization and initiation of vaccine administration.

The fourth request was for jurisdictions to decide whether to participate in the Pharmacy Partnership for Long-Term Care Program. To reduce the burden on health departments, HHS created this partnership with Walgreens and CVS to offer on-site COVID vaccination for all residents of long-term care facilities once these highly vulnerable people were recommended to receive the vaccine. The letter said that CDC would be coordinating with the jurisdictions shortly to share information on facilities interested in that service and that states could opt out of the program if they wanted to develop their own plans to vaccinate this highly prioritized population. And finally, states were told they would within a week receive additional planning estimates and scenarios to inform planning, although the estimates would not reflect any allocation decisions.

To support this level of preparedness by November 15, jurisdictions were asked to return all the requested information to CDC by November 2 (i.e., within one week), including (1) a signed DUA, (2) identification of up to five priority Phase 1 sites with ultracold storage capacity, (3) enrollment data for Phase 1 providers (for up to five sites, as prioritized), (4) enrollment of Phase 1 providers in VTrckS (again, for up to five sites, as prioritized), and (5) notification of whether the jurisdiction was opting out of the long-term care pharmacy program with CVS and Walgreens.

After canvassing her membership, Claire Hannan summarized the collective unease caused by these requests. "How could states allow vaccine to be sent to administration sites before it is approved or recommended, and before these sites are adequately trained on storage and handling?" she asked in an October 2020 internal communication to Association of Immunization Managers. "Most immunization program managers (PMs) don't even fully understand the storage and handling requirements themselves yet, so they are not in a position to trust facilities to store it correctly. In addition, PMs don't have a good grasp of expected supply and how that supply will be allocated. So committing supply at this point to five sites without understanding the overall supply and allocation strategy is difficult" (Claire Hannan, internal communication to Association of Immunization Managers, October 2020). Despite the significant concerns, most states were able to eventually supply CDC with the requested information. Although not all states met the deadline, most were able to respond within the requested time frame or ask for additional consultation with the CDC to clarify outstanding concerns.

During the home stretch of the vaccine development phase, it became clear that vaccines would not be approved by Election Day, yet the president's promises continued.

"We will deliver 100 million doses of a safe vaccine before the end of the year,"[22] he told a campaign rally on October 26 in Allentown, Pennsylvania, "and maybe quite a bit sooner than that." The bold predictions from the nation's chief executive officer compared to the silence on potential allocation numbers from the CDC to the states did not go unnoticed. Nor did the disregard for one of the top lessons from the H1N1 flu vaccine rollout in 2009: when predictions on timing and amount of vaccine availability did not match reality, the credibility of all levels of government was diminished. The run-up to the COVID vaccine rollout in 2020 left many among those who had responded to H1N1 in 2009 with an eerie sense of déjà vu.

Amid a global pandemic, American voters went to the polls on Tuesday, November 3. However, because of the time needed to count so many mail-in ballots, Joe Biden was not declared the winner until three days after, on November 6. Three days after that, on November 9, at 6:45 a.m., Pfizer and BioNTech issued a press release that truly sent shock waves around the world.

"Today is a great day for science and humanity. The first set of results from our Phase 3 COVID-19 vaccine trial provides the initial evidence of our vaccine's ability to prevent COVID-19,"[23] declared Dr. Albert Bourla, Pfizer chairman and CEO. "With today's news," he continued, "we are a significant step closer to providing people around the world with a much-needed breakthrough to help bring an end to this global health crisis." Clinical data demonstrated that Pfizer's two-dose, mRNA vaccine had a remarkable 90%-plus vaccine efficacy in preventing COVID. Amid this news, jurisdictions made their final preparations to get shots in arms and start the historic race to vaccinate America.

REFERENCES

1. Levins H. Inside the complexity of COVID vaccine distribution. University of Pennsylvania, Leonard Davis Institute for Health Economics. December 5, 2020. Available at: https://ldi .upenn.edu/our-work/research-updates/inside-the-complexity-of-covid-vaccine-distribution. Accessed September 14, 2022.

2. Cohen E, Bonifield J, Jenkins S. Pfizer's ultra-cold vaccine, a "very complex" distribution plan and an exploding head emoji. *CNN*. November 11, 2020. Available at: https://edition.cnn.com/ 2020/11/10/health/pfizer-vaccine-distribution-cold-chain/index.html. Accessed September 12, 2022.

3. Centers for Disease Control and Prevention. COVID-19 vaccination program interim playbook for jurisdiction operations. Version 1.0, September 16, 2020. Available at: https://stacks .cdc.gov/view/cdc/93806. Accessed September 12, 2022.

4. US Department of Health and Human Services. From the factory to the frontlines: the Operation Warp Speed strategy for distributing a COVID-19 vaccine. Available at: https:// www.hhs.gov/sites/default/files/strategy-for-distributing-covid-19-vaccine.pdf. Accessed September 14, 2022.

5. Association of State and Territorial Health Officials. Leading health organizations unite to implement national COVID-19 vaccination plan. October 20, 2020. Available at: https://www .astho.org/communications/newsroom/older-releases/leading-health-organizations-unite-implement-national-covid-19-vaccination-plan. Accessed September 14, 2022.

6. Branswell H. Confusion spreads over system to determine priority access to Covid-19 vaccines. *STAT*. July 22, 2020. Available at: https://www.statnews.com/2020/07/22/confusion-spreads-over-system-to-determine-priority-access-to-covid-19-vaccines. Accessed September 14, 2022.

7. National Academies of Sciences, Engineering, and Medicine. *Framework for Equitable Allocation of COVID-19 Vaccine*. Washington, DC: National Academies Press; 2020. https://doi .org/10.17226/25917.

8. Sekar K. Immunization information systems: overview and current issues, February 2022. Congressional Research Service. February 1, 2022. Available at: https://crsreports.congress .gov/product/pdf/R/R47024. Accessed September 22, 2022.

9. Bajak A, Heath D. A national system to prioritize COVID-19 vaccines has largely failed as states rely on their own systems. *USA Today*. Updated March 3, 2021. Available at: https:// www.usatoday.com/story/news/investigations/2021/03/03/covid-19-vaccine-distribution-system-fails-live-up-promise/6878303002. Accessed September 14, 2022.

10. LaFraniere S. Trump health aide pushes bizarre conspiracies and warns of armed revolt. *New York Times*. September 14, 2020. Available at: https://www.nytimes.com/2020/09/14/us/politics/caputo-virus.html. Accessed September 12, 2022.

11. Centers for Disease Control and Prevention. COVID-19 vaccination program operational guidance. Available at: https://www.cdc.gov/vaccines/covid-19/covid19-vaccination-guidance .html. Accessed September 14, 2022.

12. Routh J. COVID-19 vaccine implementation planning update. Centers for Disease Control and Prevention. October 30, 2020. Available at: https://www.cdc.gov/vaccines/acip/meetings/downloads/slides-2020-10/COVID-Routh-508.pdf. Accessed August 13, 2022.

13. Bourla A. *Moonshot: Inside Pfizer's Nine-Month Race to Make the Impossible Possible*. [Kindle edition]. New York, NY: Harper Business; 2022.

14. National Archives and Records Administration. Remarks by President Trump on vaccine development. May 15, 2020. Available at: https://trumpwhitehouse.archives.gov/briefings-statements/remarks-president-trump-vaccine-development. Accessed September 14, 2022.

15. Factbase. Remarks: Donald Trump holds a virtual Arizona tele-rally—July 18, 2020. [Transcript]. July 18, 2020. Available at: https://factba.se/transcript/donald-trump-remarks-tele-rally-arizona-july-18-2020. Accessed September 14, 2022.

16. Centers for Disease Control and Prevention. CDC COVID-19 vaccination planning: August letter to health departments. August 4, 2020.

17. Herper M, Florko N. Drug makers rebut Trump tweet that FDA "deep state" is delaying Covid-19 vaccines and drugs. *STAT*. August 22, 2020. Available at: https://www.statnews .com/2020/08/22/drug-makers-rebut-trump-tweet-that-fda-deep-state-delaying-covid19-vaccines-drugs. Accessed September 14, 2022.

18. National Archives and Records Administration. Remarks by President Trump in press briefing, September 18, 2020. September 18, 2020. https://trumpwhitehouse.archives.gov/briefings-statements/remarks-president-trump-press-briefing-september-18-2020. Accessed September 14, 2022.

19. New York State. National Governors Association submits list of questions to Trump administration on effective implementation of COVID-19 vaccine. October 18, 2020. Available at: https://www.governor.ny.gov/news/national-governors-association-submits-list-questions-trump-administration-effective. Accessed September 14, 2022.

20. US Department of Health and Human Services. Answers to National Governors Association questions on vaccine distribution and planning. Available at: https://www.hhs.gov/sites/default/files/national-governors-association-questions-on-vaccine-distribution-planning.pdf. Accessed September 14, 2022.

21. Centers for Disease Control and Prevention. CDC vaccination planning: October letter to health departments. October 26, 2020.

22. Rev. Donald Trump rally speech transcript. Allentown, PA. October 26, 2020. Available at: https://www.rev.com/blog/transcripts/donald-trump-rally-speech-transcript-allentown-pa-october-26. Accessed September 14, 2022.

23. Pfizer. Pfizer and BioNTech announce vaccine candidate against COVID-19 achieved success in first interim analysis from phase 3 study. November 9, 2020. Available at: https://www.pfizer.com/news/press-release/press-release-detail/pfizer-and-biontech-announce-vaccine-candidate-against. Accessed September 14, 2022.

6

Shots in Arms

With COVID, the situation is we know that if you're vaccinated and up to date with your vaccinations, you have a 90% reduction in the risk of death. If you are unlucky enough to get infected . . . another 90% reduction would be anti-virals . . . Almost no one in this country should be dying from COVID, if we were up to date on our vaccinations and got appropriate anti-viral treatment.[1]

–Robert Califf, FDA Commissioner, May 7, 2022

I would recommend it. And I would recommend it to a lot of people that don't want to get it and a lot of those people voted for me, frankly. But again, we have our freedoms and we have to live by that and I agree with that also. But it is a great vaccine. It is a safe vaccine and it is something that works.[2]

–Former President Trump in a *Fox News* interview, March 16, 2021

In the spring of 2020, Sandra Lindsay was working as the director of critical care nursing at Long Island Jewish Medical Center in Queens, New York.[3] An immigrant from Jamaica, she earned both a bachelor's and a master's degree in nursing. She rose through the ranks and, at the outset of the COVID pandemic, was managing a team of hundreds of nurses caring for critically ill COVID patients. That spring, her hospital had tripled its intensive care capacity to about 150 beds to care for the waves of people suffering from a disease that had been completely unknown just months earlier. She had seen firsthand the devastation caused by COVID.

At 9:20 a.m. on the cold morning of December 14, 2020, Sandra Lindsay became the first person in the United States to publicly receive a coronavirus vaccination outside of a clinical trial. "I hope this marks the beginning of the end to a very painful time in our history,"[4] she told reporters as the first public COVID-19 vaccination was live-streamed and broadcast around the world. At the time of her vaccination, 292,398 Americans had died of COVID-related illness.[5] It had been a painful time indeed.

Planning that led up to that day had been intense and contentious. The hours put in by thousands of public health professionals had been long and sometimes brutal. The speed of decision-making and the thousands of details that needed to be addressed to get shots in arms was dizzying. Misinformation and conspiracy theories about the vaccine had already been spreading rapidly through social media and were highly concerning. And yet, despite all the challenges encountered and surmounted to get to launch day, the reality of finally beginning to deliver and administer a vaccine to beat back the worst pandemic in a century was exhilarating.

The day before the first COVID shot was administered outside of a clinical trial, the leadership of the Association of Immunization Managers (AIM) sent a message to its membership that framed this critical turning point in the fight against COVID. "Today is a momentous day," the message began. "Now your work truly enters the spotlight. For over eleven months, you have waited, and hoped, and planned—and now is the time to put those plans into action" (AIM internal communication, December 13, 2020). In this message, AIM leaders acknowledged the hard but historic work that preceded the launch:

> We know you are fatigued from the planning process you have gone through these past months. We know you may be feeling the same lack of appreciation or even hostility that many of our colleagues have endured simply for doing their job. But now is the time to charge forward with what we have been saying all along will likely be the greatest public health effort of our generation. We are SO PROUD to be a part of this effort with you. And indeed, we are about to make history!

The message captured what was unique about this vaccine campaign and anticipated what would lie ahead, stating:

> What we are embarking upon is unprecedented. Never in human history has a nation set out to vaccinate nearly their entire population in such a short period of time. The challenge is immense, the complexity is daunting, and none of us are under the illusion that this will be easy. We know you will likely encounter trials ahead, some predictable and some unknown. And we know you will confront them with the problem-solving acumen and can-do attitude that honors our training as public health professionals and pervades our field. There may likely be the need for course corrections, and if so, we will change what is in our power to change, and we will do it together.

The communication closed with a message from the prominent leader of a previous battle that closely resembled the sentiments shared by nurse Sandra Lindsay: "On such an occasion it does not seem improper to quote Winston Churchill. At a turning point early in World War II, he famously said, 'Now this is not the end. It is not even the beginning of the end. But perhaps it is the end of the beginning'" (AIM internal communication, December 13, 2020).

THE FIRST WEEKS

In the first week of the vaccination campaign, 2.8 million doses of COVID vaccine were administered. By the end of March 2021, the nation's public health system had distributed 180.6 million total doses.[6(p33)] Never in American history had so many vaccines been delivered and administered in such a short time. The sense of relief and joy among the first to be vaccinated was palpable. The fast action to protect those most vulnerable and on the front lines was a triumph. Three vaccine products were eventually authorized by the Food and Drug Administration (FDA) for use on an emergency basis: Pfizer's (Comirnaty) on December 11, 2020; Moderna's (*Spikevax*) on December 18, 2020; and Janssen/Johnson & Johnson's COVID vaccine on February 27, 2021.

However, in those early days, the number of vaccine doses distributed to jurisdictions and federal partners varied significantly from week to week as a result of manufacturer supply. These changes complicated jurisdictions' ability to plan effectively and communicate realistic expectations to the public. They also raised questions about how to address vaccine supply needed for second-dose administration of the two-dose schedule.

A major revision in the total vaccine available to ship in the first week of the rollout contributed to public confusion when Operation Warp Speed (OWS) leaders unexpectedly reduced the estimates previously provided to states for their second-week allocations. They had originally estimated 7.3 million doses would be available but drastically downgraded the allocations when only about 4.3 million shots turned out to be ready to ship. The discrepancy left many governors infuriated as public health officials scrambled to revise their vaccination plans and had to communicate their change of plans to a highly anxious public.

Although never fully explained, the reduced allocations seemed to revolve around an FDA requirement for companies to complete a certificate of analysis for each product at least 48 hours before the vaccine was distributed. To his credit, General Gus Perna accepted full responsibility for the change, stating, "It was a planning error, and I am responsible."[7] Striking a theme that would dominate the campaign for the next few months, he added, "We're learning from it. We're trying to get better."[7]

Coming so early in the rollout, this bump heightened anxiety among jurisdictions about the difficulty in executing a plan without reliable estimates of vaccine supply. The early troubles were reflected in public polling conducted by the Gallup organization, which reported that in January 2021 only 34% of Americans said they were satisfied or very satisfied with the vaccination process.[8] As the Biden administration took over, it announced several aggressive goals and new policies, all of which benefited from increased production over time. By the end of February, a steadily increasing cadence of vaccine deliveries became more predictable. From February 28, 2021, to March 27, 2021, the partnership distributed an average of about 21.1 million doses of the Pfizer, Moderna, and Janssen/Johnson & Johnson vaccines per week, allowing tens of millions of the most at-risk and vulnerable Americans to be protected.

As exciting as the launch had been, it did not take long for additional bumps in the rollout to emerge. Most of the earliest challenges stemmed from too little vaccine supply. One of the biggest challenges was adjusting to the reality that available vaccine supplies did not match the quantities originally projected by the Trump administration. The lack of clarity on how much vaccine would be available and when, along with the need to cancel or add vaccination clinic appointments weekly or even change clinic sites based on vaccine supply, created an early public perception that the rollout was chaotic. It was a predictable and avoidable redux of errors that had been made in the H1N1 vaccine campaign of 2009.

At the OWS launch in May 2020, Dr. Moncef Slaoui said, "I have very recently seen early data from a clinical trial with a coronavirus vaccine. And this data made me feel even more confident that we will be able to deliver a few hundred million doses of vaccine by the end of 2020."[9] In the weeks that followed, President Trump offered confident assurances about the availability of a vaccine to 100 million Americans by year's end. "We expect to have 100 million doses of vaccine available before the end of the year and maybe much sooner than that," Trump declared on July 18.[10] Adding to unreasonable expectations, White House spokesperson Brian Morgenstern repeatedly told the press that the administration was preparing to deliver vaccine "to every zip code in the United States within 24 hours of an FDA approval."[11] As the launch approached, states were asked to identify three to five sites to preposition vaccine—not nearly every zip code, but expectations had been raised.

After the election, reality set in. The White House had to significantly scale back its projections in late November and December to meet the reality of limited vaccine production. "We plan to have enough vaccine doses available for use in the US population to immunize about 20 million individuals in the month of December and another 25 to 30 million per month on an ongoing basis from thereon,"[12] Dr. Slaoui said on November 13. The shifting projections and wide variation gave the states little insight to inform their planning for the first phases of distribution.

As potential vaccine numbers changed by the thousands, states were left to guess what resources would be needed to support vaccination campaigns in their communities. "It felt like we were always behind the eight ball," recalled Alaska program director Matthew Bobo. "A lot of our planning was done in the dark" (author oral interview with Matthew Bobo, MPH, December 15, 2021). Robert Swanson from Michigan stated, "There was a gap in information up until almost the day vaccine was being distributed" (author oral interview with Robert Swanson, MPH, December 15, 2021). Brian Tyler, the CEO of McKesson Corporation, which is the largest distributor of vaccines in the United States, summarized it this way: "We were building plans for unknown vaccines, manufactured by unknown manufacturers, in unknown quantities, approved to be administered in unknown patient populations. I think at one time we had 39 or 49 scenarios going for how we would build out our facilities."[13]

In addition to unrealistic expectations about supply, one of the other major challenges that emerged in the early days of the vaccine rollout was understanding and communicating the reporting gap in doses delivered versus doses administered as reported by the states, clinicians, and pharmacy partners in the Centers for Disease Control and

Prevention (CDC) vaccine tracker. At any given time, the quantity of vaccine in a state could be far higher than the doses administered as a result of the lag time between delivery and clinicians giving shots. However, given the short supply of vaccines, many were critical of what looked like states' delaying vaccination or "hoarding" vaccines.[14] In retrospect, this issue stemmed in part from a failure by program leaders to anticipate how the reporting of both numbers—vaccines distributed and vaccines administered—would be perceived by the public and the media and how not educating the public before the rollout on the reasons that might cause such a gap would be a problem.

These reasons were primarily operational and not related to hoarding; they included the need for some jurisdictions to take time to break down large vaccine shipments into smaller batches that could be redistributed around the state. As well, they involved the delays in operationalizing new scheduling systems, the challenges in ensuring that enough patients could be organized for a clinic before vaccine vials were opened to reduce waste, and the need to rely on third-party vaccine administrators who had to set up their operations in support of the campaign. Added to these complications were that the vaccine rollout started just before end-of-year holidays and there were thus potential delays in reporting on vaccine administration. The delay between vaccine delivery and administration also reflected that earlier in the summer CDC officials had such a difficult time educating the OWS leadership on the essential difference between vaccine distribution and vaccine administration. Despite these reasons, some press outlets pointed to the gap to insinuate that the delay resulted from a planning failure on the part of OWS and the states and sharply criticized their vaccine administration performance.

A WHIRLWIND OF EARLY POLICY CHANGES

This situation unfolded against a backdrop of post-holiday surges in COVID case counts and deaths, which increased the urgency of vaccination. Trump administration officials fielded sharp questions from the public and the press, who wanted to know why vaccine administration in the states was so "slow."[15,16,17] In response, the federal government initiated three significant changes in the early days of the rollout that upended prior planning. Each change contributed further to a perceived lack of coordination between the federal government and the states. These three policy changes were (1) early expansion of the recommended target priority group beyond the initial CDC's Advisory Committee on Immunization Practice (ACIP) recommendation to increase the number of individuals eligible, (2) a change in the federal management of second-dose reserves, and (3) a proposed but never implemented change in vaccine allocation related to vaccine administration performance. Each of these policies caused considerable anxiety but also admirable adaptability among the jurisdictions.

The policy changes were announced by Secretary Azar at a press conference on January 12, 2021,[18] just six days after the violent riot in the US Capitol by pro-Trump supporters trying to block the certification of election results and eight days before President-Elect Biden's inauguration. The first announcement focused on vaccine prioritization and who should get vaccinated first. In early December 2020, ACIP recommended to Dr. Redfield, the CDC director, that those who should receive vaccines in the initial phase of the vaccination program, dubbed Phase 1A, be health care personnel and residents of long-term care facilities. Subsequently, on December 20 and 21, 2020, ACIP met again and recommended that after Phase 1A, vaccination should be offered in a Phase 1B to persons age 75 and older and non-health care frontline essential workers, and then, in Phase 1C, to persons age 65 to 74 years, persons age 16 to 64 with high-risk medical conditions, and other essential workers. Dr. Redfield adopted both recommendations for priority groups.

States appreciated the phased recommendations, which were mostly adopted with little variation. However, in retrospect, a key element initially missing from the conversation was guidance on how and when a state should make the transition to Phase 1B: Should it be when all those in 1A who wanted to be vaccinated were? How long is it reasonable to keep those who also badly wanted the vaccine and were at high risk for infection or severe disease waiting? In the rush to prioritize limited supply, little consideration was given to the pivot point in terms of when to move to the next phase.

To address the situation, Secretary Azar announced at the same January 12, 2021, press conference that jurisdictions should essentially skip the planned move to Phase 1B and open vaccination to all eligible persons age 65 and older and to all people under age 65 with a documented comorbidity. The announcement instantly spurred questions among the state and local programs about how this expansion might open the floodgates wider than anticipated and divert vaccine away from the most vulnerable patients. It also spurred questions about what states and vaccine clinics should use as documentation to verify such comorbidities and what would be the process to review and approve these attestations.

Furthermore, Secretary Azar appeared to blame state programs for vaccinating according to prior plans and following guidance that was developed by OWS and his own agency, the Department of Health and Human Services (HHS). "Some states' heavy-handed micromanagement of this process has stood in the way of vaccines reaching a broader swath of the vulnerable population more quickly,"[18] the secretary stated. His comments reflected a sharp shift in tone from earlier statements about how the OWS purpose was to support governors' plans and how distribution decisions would be locally executed. Just four weeks into the nascent rollout, conditions set in advance to help support a managed rollout began to be thrown out the window.

The second major change announced by Secretary Azar dealt with alterations in federal management of vaccines for second doses. Second-dose administration and allocation and ordering was complicated for many reasons. For example, not everyone would return to the same location for the second dose, and not all would return for a second dose if they had significant side effects or hesitancy after their first dose. Some health officials even debated the merits of giving a first dose to more people and then delaying a second dose for several months, a strategy proposed for use in the United Kingdom, with the reasoning that more "first jabs" will help protect more people until vaccine supplies increased.[19]

At a December 2, 2020, prelaunch press conference, General Perna stated that the federal government would hold back the second dose of vaccine to jurisdictions to make sure that enough vaccine doses would be available for people to receive their second dose at the appropriate time, explaining:

> We are going to send half the doses based on allocations to the jurisdictions and agencies, because it is a two dose regimen, as Dr. Slaoui just talked about, so half of the allocation will be sent out and then 21 days later for Pfizer and 28 days later for Moderna, we send out the second half of allocations. Two reasons, one, to ensure that we don't over administer and that we have the second dose on hand. And second reason is to make sure that we don't overwhelm limited storage capability and capacity at the state level. We want to augment their plans, enable their plans, not constrain them from the greatest distribution capability that they have. We utilize a Tiberius platform that we developed, which is a capability that takes in all the informative data from the states, hospitals, doctor's offices, pharmacies.[20]

At a press conference one week later, an OWS official reiterated that the federal government would set aside some vaccine doses from the initial total supply as part of a reserve. He said that as the federal government became more confident in the manufacturing process, the plan would transition to a smaller reserve of vaccine doses and increase state allocations.[6(p40)]

However, at the same January 12, 2021, press conference at which he announced the expansion of priority groups, Secretary Azar said:

> We're now making the full reserve of doses we have available for order . . . we had always planned to move to a more advanced phase of how we manage this. Once we had confidence in our supply chains, that is the key trigger we needed to see. Because we now have a consistent pace of production, we can now ship all of the doses that had been held in physical reserve with second doses being supplied by doses coming off of manufacturing lines with quality control.[18]

The rationale was that this move would free up vaccine being held back for second doses and lead to more first-dose administration. Indeed, Secretary Azar's statement caused many state health officials to anticipate receiving a larger weekly allocation of vaccine for first doses as second-dose inventory would be released. But the mentioned cache of reserve doses that states thought were being held back did not actually exist: there was no warehouse full of vaccines waiting for shipment in three or four weeks.

At the end of December, the federal government had already begun shipping all doses and holding back none.[21] Second-dose inventory was being shipped along with first doses.

After several days of confusion, on January 15, Secretary Azar walked back his earlier statement and confirmed that the federal government did not have a stockpile of reserved second doses of vaccine. There would be no immediate hoped-for boost in supply. Dr. Nirav Shah, the state health officer for Maine and president of the Association of State and Territorial Health Officials (ASTHO) at the time explained the situation's impact to his state this way: "Who is in line will not change. The velocity of that line will change because this bolus of doses that we intuited was coming based on Azar's comments is not coming."[21]

A third announced change represented perhaps the biggest deviation from what jurisdictions had previously been told about how vaccines would be allocated among the states. Prelaunch, jurisdictions were informed that after considering several options, OWS had agreed to utilize the same system that had been used by CDC for H1N1 vaccines in 2009 in which allocations were issued pro rata according to jurisdictions' adult populations. However, in response to reports showing substantial variability in the gap between vaccines delivered and vaccines administered among the states, Secretary Azar announced a new policy. On January 12, 2021, he said:

> Effective two weeks from now, we are changing how we allocate first doses among the states, in order to ensure doses are being put to use and put to use for the most vulnerable. We will be allocating them based on the pace of administration as reported by states and by the size of the 65 and over population in each state. We're giving States two weeks' notice of this shift to give them the time necessary to plan and to improve their reporting if they think their data is faulty.[18]

He added, "This new system gives states a strong incentive to ensure that all vaccinations are being promptly reported, which they're currently not. And it gives states a strong incentive, ensure doses are going to work, protecting people rather than sitting on shelves or in freezers."[18] Implying that states were not doing all they could to vaccinate America and instead were allowing vaccine to sit unused and then announcing such a significant and punitive policy change just days before the Trump administration was about to leave office was maddening to many public health officials. It reflected a complete lack of appreciation for the reasons why vaccine administration rates were lower than vaccines shipped; it failed to account for the diverse systems states were employing to distribute vaccines along with pharmacy partners; and it blamed states for the performance of a vast network of vaccination sites, including hospitals and health centers, many of which were in rural areas with limited support to stand-up clinics. In the end, the Biden team never implemented this allocation change when the team took over days later.

The day before the outgoing administration announced policy changes intended to speed up vaccine administration, the CDC published an annex to its playbook that included new detailed guidance for jurisdictions.[22] Coming nearly a month after the launch of the program, the release reinforced the proverbial "building the plane while you are flying it" orientation that characterized planning delays in the summer of 2020. The guidance issued urgently needed considerations regarding how and when to transition from vaccinating initial populations to increasing shots among additional priority populations. Additional guidance focused on further prioritizing while balancing access and demand, developing strategies to reach critical populations, increasing vaccine confidence, and leveraging additional public-private partnerships—all items that would have alleviated a great deal of criticism and delay had they been cleared and shared prior to the vaccine launch.

Indeed, the Trump administration's response to criticism of the slow pace of the initial rollout further reveals a lack of attention to and confusion over the role of states. On December 30, 2020, President Trump responded to criticism that the vaccine rollout was moving too slowly. "The Federal Government has distributed the vaccines to the states," the president stated in a tweet, "Now it is up to the states to administer. Get moving!"[23]

The tweet is fascinating on several levels. First, it reflects the president's predictable strategy throughout the pandemic of shifting blame and avoiding accountability. Second, it captures the critical difference between delivering and administering vaccine that was never fully understood or explicit in OWS structure and planning. Third, it reflects the president's fundamental misunderstanding about the distribution plan. While the president notably blames the states in this tweet, on numerous previous occasions he said that the military would be "totally involved" in vaccine distribution; meanwhile, the OWS brass led by General Perna and Paul Mango were touting that the private sector would have the lead in distribution. Former secretary of defense Mark Esper provides this candid admission in his memoir:

> Contrary to what the president was saying publicly, though, the DoD [Department of Defense] was not going to be part of the distribution system. General Perna was telling me that, barring some type of emergency, he was "100% confident that DoD will not be part of the distribution." It wasn't that the DoD couldn't do this or opposed doing so. We just wanted to use the established logistical network of the commercial sector that reached all across and in every nook and cranny of America. In addition, it was a good way to prime the economy and get people back to work. I tried to clarify that with the president on a few occasions, but it never seemed to stick. Later in the summer, I would become concerned that the media would focus in on this contradiction and ask me to somehow explain the president's misstatements.[24(p285)]

It seems that when the going got rough, the OWS leaders couldn't decide which direction to point the finger of blame.

Finally, the president's tweet provides a clear rebuttal to Paul Mango's assertion just nine days earlier that "the only thing [the states] really have to do is tell us where they want things shipped and everything is shipped there."[25] It was also Mango who told us, "The army guys firmly believed that the private sector could perform this a lot better than the public sector—I'm talking about distribution and administration—and they did so almost flawlessly" (author oral interview with Paul Mango, MBA, December 13, 2021). Finally, according to Mango, after OWS directed nearly $30 billion of taxpayer funds to private corporations to develop and distribute vaccines but next to nothing to state and local governments to administer them, the OWS response to the CDC request for state and local funds was as follows: "We were like, 'Guys, we can't . . . we're resource constrained here.'"

While Paul Mango was both publicly and privately dismissive of the need to fund state and local jurisdictions, Dr. Slaoui further demonstrated the lack of agreement on this critical issue among top OWS leaders. During an interview on January 15, 2021, in the chaotic early days of the rollout, when asked by the *Washington Post* what OWS could have done the year before to pave the way for getting the vaccine into arms, he responded:

> What we have discussed at length with each department of health in the states was their need to tell us where to send the vaccine . . . I think now, looking backwards, we could have been more specific into the discussion around what resources [states] may need to actually deliver those vaccine doses into the arms from the moment they have been delivered to them.[26]

It was a refreshing moment of candor, but Dr. Slaoui was seemingly unaware of the funding requests from the National Governors Association (NGA) and from ASTHO, AIM, and others, along with Mango's veto of the CDC's budget request. Dr. Slaoui then suggested states had never asked for resources:

> I should note that no single state has raised that question to us during the months of September, October, November, where on a weekly basis we were visiting the departments and discussing plans and how it will go . . . Gus Perna and I were always of the view that it's very hard for anyone centrally to know there would be 2,000 people to vaccinate at this particular hospital or center. That is information that is understood by each state and each county. It's possible there was [a financial] issue, but frankly it was never raised to us.[26]

But it was raised repeatedly, and as previously noted, the first six questions the NGA publicly had submitted to OWS in October all prioritized funding.[27] Demonstrating the complete misunderstanding between federal and state leaders, the official response from HHS to the NGA's inquiry was frustrating: "In considering funding needs, states should recognize that most of the major costs of a vaccine campaign are already being covered."[28]

Despite the confusion among OWS leaders, the first $3 billion to support state and local activities to administer COVID vaccination passed by Congress in December 2020 was finally awarded to the 64 state and local jurisdictions on January 18, 2021, more than a month after the first vaccines arrived.[29] And even though grants were made by January 18, the award notice required jurisdictions to submit detailed work plans and budgets addressing 35 required activities within 45 days of receipt. This meant that the public officials supporting the front lines of vaccine distribution were being asked to essentially shift their focus from distributing vaccines to filling out grant requests. This was all work that could have been completed the previous summer had there been advance agreement on the resource needs for a successful campaign at the federal, state, and local levels. Instead, the OWS leadership's ideological preference for the private over the public sector, until overridden by Congress, created yet another avoidable bottleneck in the critical first months of vaccine distribution.

MORE VACCINES AND PHARMACY CAPACITY ADDED TO THE FIGHT

On December 18, 2020, just four days after the first Pfizer shots were given, the FDA's Vaccines and Related Biological Products Advisory Committee approved Moderna's COVID vaccine for emergency use in individuals age 18 and over. A few days later, the first COVID vaccine doses were distributed through CDC's Pharmacy Partnership for Long-Term Care Program. As part of the overall nationwide vaccination strategy, CDC developed the Pharmacy Partnership program to provide all long-term care settings an option to enroll in this program. The CDC engaged retail pharmacy partners CVS and Walgreens to secure vaccine and provide on-site vaccination of residents, at no cost to the facility. This program was designed to provide end-to-end management of the COVID-19 vaccination process, including storage, handling, cold chain management, on-site vaccinations, and fulfillment of reporting requirements to facilitate safe and effective vaccination of this patient population while reducing the burden on facilities and health departments.

The Federal Retail Pharmacy Program (FRPP), which launched on February 9, 2021, was another strategy to quickly vaccinate the nation. The FRPP, not to be confused with the CDC's Pharmacy Partnership for Long-Term Care Program, was "designed to use the strength and expertise of pharmacy partners to help rapidly vaccinate the American public."[30] It built upon both the positive experience of utilizing pharmacies as vaccination sites for H1N1 influenza in 2009 and data showing that over 90% of Americans live within five miles of a pharmacy. Through this program, enrolled retail pharmacies nationwide would receive COVID-19 vaccine supply directly from the federal government, not from state allocation channels. As the supply of vaccine increased, so would the number of retail locations that provided COVID-19 vaccination. Pharmacy partners signed agreements to use this supply to vaccinate eligible individuals at no cost to the patients. The program relied on collaboration with public health agencies to encourage individuals to go to pharmacies to get vaccinated, and over time this approach proved to be an indispensable part of the overall national strategy.

Within the first year, a total of 21 retail pharmacy partners, including long-term care pharmacies—with more than 41,000 locations online—were participating in the program and administering doses nationwide. And as of June 8, 2022, retail pharmacies across the United States reported that more than 254.3 million doses had been administered, which included eight million doses administered on-site to long-term care facilities in the early days of the vaccination program.[31] This total represents approximately 43% of all COVID vaccine doses administered in the United States—an exceptional achievement based on an extraordinary partnership. But as convenient as pharmacies are to most people, some areas of the country have no pharmacy close by.

An *ABC News* analysis of pharmacy locations across the country revealed that 150 counties have no pharmacy and that nearly 4.8 million people live in a county where there is only one pharmacy for every 10,000 residents or more.[31] Public health agencies aware of such gaps in their jurisdictions acted to fill in capacity where necessary. Moreover, with less than half of all COVID vaccinations taking place in pharmacies, this approach illustrates the shortsightedness of the OWS planners who initially pushed aside the CDC recommendation to use an array of providers from across the public and private sectors.

AN UNPRECEDENTED TRANSITION

The baton of national leadership for the COVID vaccination campaign was handed to a new administration when Joe Biden was inaugurated the 46th president of the United States on January 20, 2021. Even before inauguration day, Biden signaled a collaborative, science-informed approach to battling the pandemic. On November 9, 2020, the president-elect announced a 12-member COVID Advisory Board charged with crafting a plan to curb the rapidly spreading virus.

The group was cochaired by former surgeon general Dr. Vivek Murthy, former FDA commissioner Dr. David Kessler, and Dr. Marcella Nunez-Smith of Yale University. To the relief of long-ignored state and local public health officials, it included members with high-level experience in state and local public health agencies, including Dr. Michael Osterholm, former state epidemiologist for Minnesota, and Dr. Julie Morita, former commissioner of the Chicago Department of Health. "Dealing with the coronavirus pandemic is one of the most important battles our administration will face, and I will be informed by science and by experts," Biden said in announcing his task force.[32] "The advisory board will help shape my approach to managing the surge in reported infections; ensuring vaccines are safe, effective, and distributed efficiently, equitably, and free;

and protecting at-risk populations."[32] The board's formation was announced the same day that Pfizer injected great hope around the globe by announcing its coronavirus vaccine was more than 90% effective in preventing COVID.

The White House COVID Task Force, along with the broader Biden transition team, began assessing the vaccine distribution plan from the outgoing Trump administration. Offering a breath of fresh air to public health leaders, Biden administration transition officials almost immediately began outreach to the national public health associations long shunned by the Trump officials. Channels of communication were opened to share perspectives on what was going well and where course corrections were urgently needed. For many public health officials, it was the first time they felt they had a meaningful forum to share feedback and recommendations in a spirit of partnership.

Describing how the tone changed with the turnover of administrations, in our March 17, 2022, oral interview, Claire Hannan, MPH, told us, "I distinctly recall them acknowledging the challenges communicating with the prior administration. [They said,] 'This isn't gonna happen with our administration. We're gonna communicate with you. You're gonna be at the table and we can't believe how you've been treated. And we would never ask you to do things without giving you money.'" But this fresh approach was partially undermined by a continuation of the policy of not engaging in predecisional consultation with jurisdictions. Hannan said, "I think that in their effort to not have leaks, they just didn't give out some information. [In some instances, there was] no coordination because they didn't want things to be leaked." She continued:

> The Biden team was very goal-oriented, and they immediately put out the goal of doing a hundred million shots in a hundred days. And they were big on federal solutions. I mean, they really weren't going to leave things just to the states. We thought what we were doing was working, but that wasn't enough for President Biden. He wanted more. And he basically was willing to do anything. Let's get FEMA involved, let's get the military involved, let's get the National Guard involved, let's get communities involved. Let's put out guidance. He was coming at it from every angle. And I think ultimately it was appreciated by the states, but I think it was a little stressful at first. (author oral interview with Claire Hannan, MPH, March 17, 2022)

On January 21, 2021, one day after the Biden administration had taken office, the White House released the *National Strategy for the COVID-19 Response and Pandemic Preparedness*.[33] It was a comprehensive plan focused on restoring trust and supporting "aggressive, safe, and effective vaccination campaign."[33(p4)] It set an ambitious vaccination target of administering 100 million shots within the first 100 days. Striving to highlight what would be different from the previous administration, the Biden *National Strategy* set the tone for cooperation and a laser focus on equity from the outset. And in perhaps the biggest break from the Trump OWS leaders, the plan fully embraced the need to adequately fund critical public health partners, stating, "Central to this effort will be additional support and funding for state, local, tribal, and territorial governments."[33(p8)]

Beyond the welcome change in tone, however, the plan contained several actions that the Trump administration had already implemented or had been planning to put in place shortly. For instance, the Biden *National Strategy* stated, "In order to expand the supply available to states, the administration will end the policy of holding back significant levels of doses, instead holding back a small reserve and monitoring supply to ensure that everyone receives the full regimen as recommended by the FDA."[33(p9)] This echoed what Secretary Azar had already announced a few weeks earlier. "The United States will accelerate the pace of vaccinations," the *National Strategy* affirmed, "by encouraging states and localities to move through the priority groups more quickly—expanding access to frontline essential workers and individuals over the age of 65, while staying laser-focused on working to ensure that the highest-risk members of the public, including those in congregate facilities, can access the vaccine where and when they need it,"[33(p9)] partially echoing Secretary Azar's announcement regarding moving all jurisdictions to Americans age 65 and above.

The timing of the new administration's takeover just as vaccine manufacturing and supply was rapidly expanding also allowed the Biden administration to implement the improvements the Trump administration had planned in the original phased approach. For example, the new plan promised to improve the vaccine allocation process and provide more consistent vaccine projections to inform state planning. This would build on the groundwork the Trump team had laid in manufacturing and advanced vaccine purchase. The process was made somewhat easier by the fact that vaccine manufacturing was becoming more stable and predictable so that allocations would fluctuate less; consequently, states could have more certainty in what they would receive week to week.

In the weeks surrounding the change of administrations, an unfortunate but perhaps inevitable spat broke out over the adequacy of each team's efforts. This too may have contributed inadvertently to the politicization of the vaccine campaign. Biden's criticism of the Trump team started during the transition when he said, "The Trump administration's plan to distribute vaccines is falling behind, far behind. As I long feared and warned, the effort to distribute and administer the vaccine is not progressing as it should."[34] Biden's chief of staff Ron Klain amplified the point just four days into the new administration when he appeared on the television program *Meet the Press*. In the interview, he acknowledged some progress under President Trump and then added, "But the process to distribute the vaccine, particularly outside of nursing homes and hospitals out into the community as a whole did not really exist when we came into the White House. As everyone in America has seen, the way in which people get vaccine is chaotic. It's very limited."[35] The show broadcast results of an *NBC News* poll showing 11% of voters surveyed believed vaccine administration had been going very well. Among those who said delivery fell short, 64% blamed the federal government.[35]

It is impossible to know for sure if the initial vaccine introduction could have been less chaotic, but the reality is that in any distribution of a new vaccine, supply is likely to be limited in the initial phases. That is why it is critical to have a public, transparent, and well-publicized process to determine who will be prioritized to receive the first available doses when vaccine is ready for administration. But the Trump administration put people in charge who were not familiar with the well-established process of prioritization using the CDC's ACIP. Moreover, had the Trump administration been more effective in preparing the public for the reality of an initially constrained supply rather than stoking unrealistic expectations of 100 million doses being available in every zip code before the election, perhaps some of the harshest public opinion could have been avoided by tempering expectations rather than raising and then dashing them.

A week after taking office, President Biden tried a more nuanced message: "We want to give credit to everyone involved in this vaccine effort and the prior administration and the science community and the medical sphere . . . for getting the program off the ground. And that credit is absolutely due."[36] But then the president added pointedly, "But it's also no secret that we have recently discovered, in the final days of the transition—and it wasn't until the final days we got the kind of cooperation we needed—that once we arrived, the vaccine program is [in] worse shape than we anticipated or expected."[36]

Still, in late February, White House COVID Task Force coordinator Jeff Zients told *60 Minutes* that the real credit went to the scientists who developed the vaccines and the citizens who volunteered to participate in clinical trials.[37] "The bad news," he added, "is there really was no plan to ramp up the supply of those vaccines."[37] President Biden himself said in a February 25, 2021, speech marking the 50 millionth shot being administered in the United States:

> We're moving in the right direction, though, despite the mess we inherited from the previous administration, which left us with no real plan to vaccinate all Americans . . .
>
> And here's the deal—here's the deal: The story of this vaccination campaign is like the story of everything hard and new America does: some confusion and setbacks at the start, and then if we do the right things, we have the right plan to get things moving. That's what we're seeing right now.[38]

The criticism clearly stung former president Trump and his top aides. In an exceedingly rare post-White House comment on vaccines, the former president, banned from Twitter after the Capitol riot on January 6, 2021, released a statement saying, "I hope everyone remembers when they're getting the COVID-19 (often referred to as the China Virus) Vaccine, that if I wasn't President, you wouldn't be getting that beautiful 'shot' for 5 years, at best, and probably wouldn't be getting it at all. I hope everyone remembers!"[39] Paul Mango later added, "We're delighted that more Americans are getting the vaccine, we just don't understand why they [the Biden administration] have to celebrate it by trashing what we did."[40] Unfortunately, the "trashing" of one administration's work to highlight and sometimes inflate the accomplishments of another seems to be an inescapable part of modern partisanship.

Former secretary of defense Mark Esper, who cochaired the OWS board of directors with HHS secretary Azar, added a much more balanced assessment of the transition in his recently published memoir:

> Notwithstanding the success of OWS's vaccine development and manufacturing, there were challenges in vaccine administration and reporting, but politicians and the media exaggerated the problems in the midst of a heated, partisan, postelection transition period. Much of this was unfair to Perna, Slaoui, and all the other federal employees and military personnel at HHS and the DoD, as well as the commercial companies who worked so hard for over eight months to make OWS successful and get the American people vaccinated . . . I was disappointed that the incoming Biden team would later start saying that there was really no distribution plan at all, and that they had to start from scratch. It all seemed to be a concerted effort to tarnish and reject anything associated with the Trump administration. They tried to reset the bar very low by denigrating a lot of hard work by many good people, with the aim of coming back months later to claim victory over COVID. I guess they thought that was good politics. However, it was pure politics, and it wasn't consistent with Joe Biden's promise to bring people together and unify the nation. All it did was further divide Americans and diminish public confidence in and support for the vaccines . . . Whoever gave the president those BS talking points did not serve him well.[24(p288)]

Perhaps sensing that the administration may have gone too far with the overly harsh criticism and trying to refocus on the future, Biden advisor Andy Slavitt went to *Fox News* on March 11, 2021, to try to turn the page. Offering an olive branch, he said, "We're grateful for the work that came before us and are doing the best we can to continue it and accelerate it. I would absolutely tip my hat . . . The Trump administration made sure that we got in record time a vaccine up and out. That's a great thing and it's something we should all be excited about."[41] He then plugged an upcoming Biden speech that would celebrate the acceleration of vaccine administration and highlight activities to build on that momentum.

In the end, the controversy should have centered more on debates about the adequacy of the Trump administration plans, rather than whether a plan existed. A lot of the tension stemmed from the Biden administration's accusations that the Trump administration had no plan when instead they could have said the plan was poorly communicated, poorly coordinated, and not adequately funded. Clearly, the OWS *Factory to Frontlines* strategy, the *CDC Playbook*, and required state planning and response documents all constituted plans. However, the Trump era plans did not initially include any firm information on when vaccination would start, how many doses states should expect in their early shipments, nor how providers would be reimbursed for administration. Moreover, there was no dedicated budget to execute the plans.

"To say there wasn't planning is not accurate,"[42] Claire Hannan told PolitiFact, a nonpartisan fact-checking organization that covered the controversy. She added, "However, I don't think there was communication from the federal government about the plan, about the vision, about how things would work."[42] This lack of communication underscored the biggest disconnect and resulted in a dire lack of coordination between federal, state, and local officials.

Anticipating the need for open lines of communication in the hectic final weeks leading up to the launch in November 2020, ASTHO made another last-ditch request to establish a regular time to connect with General Perna to share perspectives from the front lines. The response from OWS demonstrated once again the complete lack of understanding of the states' critical role. In a December 2, 2020, email to James Blumenstock at ASTHO, the OWS chief of staff Colonel Eric Shirley replied:

> This is a critical time for Operation Warp Speed as we are making final preparations now to distribute tens of millions of doses of a vaccine, potentially by the end of the month, and then rapidly scale to hundreds of millions in the new year. Our leaders are fiercely focused on this life-saving mission, and any additional demands for their time will pull them away from that effort. OWS leaders are committed to transparency with the American public and value communication with critical stakeholders. In that light, Dr. Slaoui and GEN Perna continue to conduct weekly public briefings, and other OWS leaders and staff continue to regularly engage various groups, organizations and associations. At this crucial time, we cannot entertain any additional battle rhythm or regularly scheduled events to our leaders' already full calendars. (email material shared with author)

WORKING THROUGH THE WHIRLWIND

Another change the Biden administration initiated was to move the functions of OWS to two new entities within the Administration for Strategic Preparedness and Response, the Countermeasures Acceleration Group (CAG) and H-CORE, the HHS Coordination Operations and Response Element.[43] The CAG was set up to rebrand the Biden team's efforts to build on OWS's acceleration of vaccine development, manufacturing, and distribution to states and to improve vaccine administration. The administration set in motion a memorandum of understanding to transition Department of Defense (DoD) responsibilities related to OWS to the CAG. According to a later review by the Government Accounting Office, the memorandum also called for HHS and DoD to develop a joint interagency process for incorporating lessons learned from the CAG's work into HHS's continued operations and to dissolve the CAG by December 31, 2021.[44]

Meanwhile, as winter 2021 turned to spring, vaccine supply steadily increased, allocations became more predictable, and every day millions of people gained protection against death, serious illness, and hospitalization from COVID. Jurisdictions were able to reach more and more people by using every available vaccine administration channel. Michele Roberts recalled this time as a period of "continuing adjustments, and ramping and scaling" (author oral interview with Michele Roberts, MPH, MSHES, December 28, 2021).

Roberts described the state health department's initial thinking that since 99% of routine vaccines are given through private-sector partners in Washington, these would naturally be the primary channel to administer COVID vaccine. But in early January, with prompting from their governor, they realized they would need mass vaccination clinics to reach large numbers of people as quickly as possible. "And we stood them up in seven to ten days," she recounted with understandable pride (author oral interview with Michele Roberts, MPH, MSHES, December 28, 2021). On the early challenges, Claire Hannan observed:

> I think what went much better than expected was that people didn't throw in the towel in those first couple of weeks when some of what we planned really wasn't working, like sending the vaccine to large hospital systems. And I was just amazed at the response, like when there was a catastrophic failure with data systems. For example, [one state's] system completely shut down, and hundreds of people just worked around the clock to fix it . . . I remember talking to [one state program manager] where so many things had gone wrong. They might have said "I can't do this," but they just brought people in, they hired more people, they figured out how to do things differently. For example, with their data systems, they needed another one and they just built it on the fly. In another state, it was near disaster, but they just kept going. I mean, they just kept showing up to work and finding a way to do it. It was amazing. (author oral interview with Claire Hannan, MPH, March 17, 2022)

Another vaccine administration strategy the Biden administration promoted in early 2021 was community-based or mass vaccination sites and the use of mobile vaccination clinics set up through the Federal Emergency Management Agency (FEMA). Reflecting the urgency of the situation, initial guidance for utilizing FEMA resources was issued on February 4, with the first FEMA community vaccination center pilot site and Mobile Vaccination Program sites established in Oakland and Los Angeles, California, shortly thereafter on February 15.[45] While jurisdictions welcomed the infusion of additional options and resources to rapidly expand COVID vaccination sites, some states reported an initial lack of coordination, with FEMA moving to open sites in states sometimes without any notification or coordination with state efforts. In addition, the ability of states to rapidly expand vaccine availability to an increasing number of established community-based sites as supply increased limited the need to utilize FEMA resources for "pop-up" sites in their jurisdictions.

The FEMA initiative was initially proposed to support up to 100 sites.[46] However, because of diminished need, the FEMA federal community vaccination center pilot sites eventually reached only 21.[47] Nevertheless, as of May 2022, these sites had administered more than 5.1 million vaccinations.[47] In addition, 14 mobile vaccination units were operating in nine states, and two units were supporting the Indian Health Service mission to vaccinate tribal communities across the Great Plains. The mobile units had delivered more than 33,700 vaccinations. Accordingly, the FEMA program made an important but relatively modest contribution to the overall campaign, and by late June the program had ended. Regarding the effectiveness of the FEMA clinics, Claire Hannan's assessment was that they were effective:

> They worked. I mean, they got a lot of vaccine out. There are a lot of issues with the data because they were set up very quickly, but they did their job. It made a huge difference because the timing was so important. We may have vaccinated the same number of people, but they may have gotten it three weeks later, four weeks later, five weeks later—how many thousands of people would've gotten COVID and died in that period of time? That was the bridge that took us from vaccinating 1 million people a day to 3 million people a day. The timing was really important. (author oral interview with Claire Hannan, MPH, March 17, 2022)

Another milestone was reached on February 22, 2021, when the first doses were distributed through the Health Resources and Services Administration (HRSA) Community Health Center COVID-19 Vaccine Program. Driven by a commitment to help those disproportionately affected by COVID-19 and the Biden administration's explicit commitment to addressing inequity, HRSA and CDC launched a program to directly allocate COVID-19 vaccines to HRSA-supported health centers.[48] These health centers provide comprehensive primary care to the medically underserved and serve some of the most vulnerable populations in America.

The program rolled out in phases, with 250 health centers initially participating by late February. To further expand the program and accelerate the delivery of vaccines to medically underserved communities and disproportionately affected populations, HRSA and CDC eventually invited an additional 700 health centers to participate, increasing the total number of invited health centers to 950. On April 7, 2021, HRSA and CDC invited all HRSA-funded health centers and health center program look-alikes to participate in the program, increasing its reach to 1,470 health centers nationwide.

Putting a special focus on the community health center channel for vaccine distribution was critical in the quest to address inequities, as nearly 91% of health center patients are individuals or families living at or below 200% of the Federal Poverty Guidelines and nearly 62% are racial or ethnic minorities.[48] However, like the FRPP, the vaccine allocation provided for this program was separate from jurisdictions' weekly allocations. This created some challenges for states as they adjusted their strategies to accommodate the direct allocations going to health centers.

Despite the coordination challenges, there was widespread understanding and support of the federal government's prerogative to provide vaccines directly to health centers to increase access to vaccines for the providers serving the nation's underserved communities and disproportionately affected populations. By June of 2021, these health centers had administered close to 21 million vaccine doses, and nearly 70% of the recipients were low-income and uninsured racial or ethnic minorities.[49] The program was a critical factor in the multifaceted strategy for closing glaring inequities that emerged early in the overall COVID vaccine campaign.

Another potential tool to address equity and help vaccinate hard-to-reach populations emerged in late February 2021 when the Janssen/Johnson & Johnson vaccine was authorized for emergency use in individuals over age 18. Unlike the previously authorized Pfizer and Moderna vaccines, which require two doses approximately three weeks apart, the Janssen vaccine requires only one initial dose and has much easier storage and handling requirements. This raised hopes that it might be easier to serve populations who may be difficult to reach, transient, or less likely to attend follow-up appointments, such as people experiencing homelessness or people living in geographically remote areas.

However, just six weeks later, the CDC and FDA announced a recommended pause in the use of the Janssen vaccine.[50] Utilizing the network of vaccine safety monitoring systems, officials were alerted to six reported cases of a rare and severe type of blood clot in individuals after receiving a dose of this vaccine. The CDC's advisory committee ACIP quickly convened two emergency meetings to review the reported cases, and 10 days after the pause commenced, ACIP reaffirmed its interim recommendation for use of the Janssen COVID-19 vaccine in persons age ≥18 years but included a warning regarding rare clotting events after vaccination, primarily among women age 18 to 49.[51]

While the pause was lifted, the safety concerns clearly had an impact on subsequent utilization. As of December 15, 2021, among approximately 488 million COVID-19 primary series doses and 56 million COVID-19 booster doses administered, only 17 million (3.5%) and 800,000 (1.6%), respectively, were Janssen COVID-19 vaccine doses.[51] Through ongoing safety surveillance and review of reports from the Vaccine Adverse Event Reporting System, additional cases of blood clots after receipt of Janssen COVID-19 vaccine, including deaths, were identified.

On December 16, 2021, ACIP therefore held another emergency meeting to review updated data on the blood clots and an updated benefit-risk assessment. At that meeting, ACIP made a recommendation "for preferential use of mRNA COVID-19 vaccines over the Janssen COVID-19 vaccine, including both primary and booster doses administered to prevent COVID-19, for all persons age ≥18 years."[51] The revised recommendation also said, "Janssen COVID-19 vaccine may be considered in some situations, including for persons with a contraindication to receipt of mRNA COVID-19 vaccines."[51]

Some anti-vaccine critics point to these issues with the Janssen vaccine as proof that COVID vaccines are not reliably safe. However, the situation highlighted the effectiveness of America's rigorous safety monitoring systems and the value of transparency when dealing with ethically challenging issues regarding the assessment of risks and benefits. "The pause on the Janssen COVID-19 vaccine has demonstrated the strength of our nation's vaccine safety monitoring system and the transparent and careful deliberations by the ACIP should raise confidence in FDA-authorized and CDC-recommended COVID-19 vaccines," American Medical Association president Susan R. Bailey, MD, said in November 2021.[52]

Public opinion approving of the vaccine campaign improved markedly as supply increased in the first months of 2021. Overall satisfaction among American adults increased from 34% in January to 44% in February, and then it shot up to 68% by March 2021.[8] Like so much of the pandemic, levels of satisfaction also reflected partisan divisions, with Republican satisfaction dipping two percentage points in February when the Biden administration became fully in charge and then trailing the Democratic satisfaction by seven percentage points in March. While the partisan differences were clear, it is not easy to disentangle how much the increased satisfaction stemmed from improvements made by the Biden team and how much simply reflected rapidly increasing supply.

Regardless of the reasons for increased public satisfaction, the Biden administration did not rest on its laurels. Around the same time the Janssen pause was initiated in the spring of 2021, the White House and federal health agencies announced a whirlwind of significant policy changes in short succession. On March 2, 2021, for example, President Biden directed states to prioritize all educators, school staff, and childcare workers.[53] He announced a goal to provide at least one shot to every teacher, school staff member, and childcare worker by the end of March. At that time, more than 30 states had already prioritized educators as essential workers eligible for prioritized vaccine. The move to override the prioritization decisions of the remaining states reflected the national sense of urgency to return to in-person schooling.

On March 29, 2021, the White House announced via press release that 90% of adults should be eligible for vaccination by April 19, 2021, and 90% of adults should have a vaccination site within five miles of where they live.[54] At that time, 31 states had said they would open to all adults by April 19. The announcement, therefore, caught close to two dozen states off guard and required them to again adjust plans, staffing, and communications. To support the push, however, the administration also announced that it was increasing the number of pharmacies in the federal pharmacy vaccination program from 17,000 to nearly 40,000 across the country and that it would stand up a dozen more mass vaccination sites by April 19. The president also announced a welcome new effort to fund community organizations to provide transportation and assistance for the nation's most at-risk seniors and people with disabilities to enable them to access vaccines.

On April 19, Pfizer requested that the FDA amend the emergency use authorization for its vaccine to include adolescents age 12 to 15. The FDA approved the request on May 10. Thus began the important but confusing process of introducing specific vaccines to younger and younger populations as adequate safety data became available. While these steps were necessary and likely unavoidable, it led to potential confusion because providers needed to be aware of regularly shifting recommendations concerning at what age patients could receive which vaccine. It also underscored the anxiety among many parents who waited to have their entire family fully vaccinated. The last step in this process commenced on June 15, 2022, when the FDA approved and CDC subsequently recommended vaccines for children five months old and above.

In early May 2021, the White House made additional announcements responding to press accounts and widespread reporting that many people were still having difficulty finding an appointment and available place to be vaccinated. On May 1, the CDC announced a new national hotline to assist with scheduling appointments and offered additional assistance to states struggling to perfect their own scheduling systems. On May 4, the White House put forth a new bold goal and made additional efforts to make vaccination appointments more accessible. President Biden announced a goal for 70% of the US adult population to have one vaccine shot and 160 million US adults to be fully vaccinated by the Fourth of July holiday "so that life can start to look closer to normal."[55]

Describing it as the next phase of the vaccination campaign, the administration said it would "make getting vaccinated more accessible than ever before, continuing to increase people's confidence in the vaccines and ensuring that everyone is reached in the response."[56] The president announced that he was directing tens of thousands of pharmacies in the federal pharmacy vaccination program to offer walk-in appointments and redirecting FEMA resources to support more pop-up clinics, smaller community vaccination sites, and more mobile clinics. FEMA resources would also aid in shipping new allocations of the vaccine to rural health clinics across the country and providing additional funding to help communities do outreach and engagement to help get people vaccinated.

To support the Fourth of July goal, the White House announced that June would be a month of action for COVID vaccination marked by the creation or expansion of numerous partnership efforts. "Throughout the month, national organizations, local government leaders, community-based and faith-based partners, businesses, employers, social media influencers, celebrities, athletes, colleges, young people, and thousands of volunteers across the nation will mobilize to make it even easier to get vaccinated and to empower their communities to get vaccinated," the White House release said.[56] These activities included offering free childcare for individuals getting vaccinated; extended hours at pharmacies across the country every Friday in June to offer more flexible appointment availability; additional outreach through community canvassing, phone banking, text banking, and vaccination events; a We Can Do This national vaccination tour; a Mayors Challenge to Increase COVID-19 Vaccinations in cities across America;

a Shots at the Shop new initiative to engage Black-owned barbershops and beauty salons; more education by blanketing local tv and radio and social media to get Americans the facts and answer their questions; a COVID-19 College Challenge wherein colleges and universities can take a pledge and commit to taking action to get their students and communities vaccinated; and a push to publicize businesses offering incentives to customers and employees to get vaccinated.[57]

At the time these all-hands-on-deck efforts were announced, both cases and deaths were falling. By midsummer, Americans were feeling hopeful that a return to normalcy was within reach. The vaccines were demonstrating amazing effectiveness and thanks to adequate supply were widely available and free. However, as some experts had predicted, a mutation in the virus was threatening to undermine so much of the progress. On July 7, 2021, the CDC reported that the Delta variant had become the dominant strain of COVID-19 in the United States. The agency estimated that over the two weeks ending on July 3, 51.7% cases in the United States were linked to the variant first identified in India.[57] Cases shot up sharply by mid-July, and shocking numbers of preventable deaths followed closely.

The July to December 2021 Delta variant surge demonstrated the effectiveness of the vaccines but also began to reveal some of their limitations. While the vaccines remained outstandingly effective in preventing severe disease, hospitalization, and death, it was becoming increasingly evident that they were not 100% effective in stopping all transmission and "breakthrough" infection. This led to disillusionment and even cynicism about the need to be vaccinated among the population and created a messaging challenge amid the shifting scientific and popular understanding and expectations. Some individuals began to question why take the vaccine at all if breakthrough infection could take place and someone could get sick even if vaccinated. Public health officials faced an uphill battle in explaining why the protection offered through vaccination, even if one had some symptoms of COVID, was important for one's own health and the health of one's community.

Partisan differences in satisfaction with the campaign also began to diverge sharply. Gallup polling showed that Republican respondents initially had double the satisfaction level over Democrats in January when the program was launched under the Trump administration (44% vs. 22%), but by March Democratic satisfaction exceeded that of Republican respondents by seven percentage points (73% vs. 66%).[8] More troubling was the increasingly stark partisan divide in people willing to be vaccinated. While many officials planning the COVID vaccine campaign were planning from the outset to expect challenges in achieving high rates of vaccination in communities of color as a result of long-standing issues of trust and mistreatment, few predicted the breakdown that would occur along partisan political affiliation.

According to tracking conducted by the nonpartisan Kaiser Family Foundation, when asked in September of 2020 if a free vaccine were available before the election, just 4 in

10 adults (42%) said they would want to get vaccinated. But whereas half of Democrats (50%) said they would get vaccinated if a vaccine were available before the election, majorities of independents (56%) and Republicans (60%) said they would not get the vaccine.[58] As vaccine supply became abundant by the summer of 2021, individuals who identified as Republicans made up a steadily increasing share of the unvaccinated. The Kaiser Family Foundation vaccine-tracking survey showed that by April 2021, "among the 43% of adults who said at that time that they had not yet been vaccinated, about four in ten (42%) identified as Republicans or Republican-leaning independents. Six months later, in October 2021, one-quarter (27%) of US adults say they have not gotten a COVID-19 vaccine, but the unvaccinated population was now disproportionately made up of those who identify as Republican or Republican-leaning, with six in ten (60%) identifying as Republican or Republican-leaning (compared to about four in ten of the US total adult population) and just one in six (17%) calling themselves Democrats or Democratic-leaning."[59]

Despite the partisan differences in willingness to be vaccinated, most Americans were optimistic about the future of the pandemic prior to the summer 2021 Delta surge. In June 2021, a record 89% said the situation was getting better, while only 3% said it was getting worse.[60] But with the onset of rapidly increasing cases and deaths due to the new variant, just one month later, in July, more Americans told Gallup the coronavirus situation in the United States was getting worse (45%) rather than better (40%).[61] It was a dramatic turnaround that came just as President Biden was touting how 67% of adults were fully vaccinated, just short of his 70% Fourth of July goal.[62]

Momentum from the month-of-action strategies began to stall in the summer of 2021. After reaching a peak of over 3.5 million doses delivered daily in mid-April 2021, the daily rate dropped to less than 500,000 shortly after the Fourth of July. The number of unvaccinated Americans who indicated that little or nothing would change their minds began to calcify, and the partisanship around COVID vaccination became increasingly toxic. In the face of this precipitous decline, the White House responded on July 6 with a new five-point plan and a heightened presidential urging. In brief remarks at the White House, Biden highlighted that it was time to move from a focus on mass vaccination clinics where thousands could be vaccinated daily to more convenient community-based vaccination sites.

Biden also made an impassioned plea that, while well-intentioned, might have hardened some opposition. "Please get vaccinated now. It works. It's free," President Biden said. "It's never been easier, and it's never been more important. Do it now for yourself and the people you care about, for your neighborhood, for your country. It sounds corny, but it's a patriotic thing to do."[63] A former CDC official later told us that this type of encouragement was coming from the wrong messenger and was possibly counterproductive because if a president people didn't support told them to do something, they were likely to do the opposite. Instead, they suggested, a career CDC doctor in a uniform backed up by an individual's own doctor making the same encouragement would be more effective.[64]

Nevertheless, the five-point plan announced that day included a central focus on equity and acknowledged a responsibility to reach the communities hardest hit by the virus. The president highlighted a number of proposed improvements: expansion of the FRPP to 42,000 local pharmacies, shipment of vaccine to more family doctors and health care providers, and establishment of a priority to serve younger people so that adolescents age 12 to 18 could get vaccinated. Furthermore, the government and health authorities would work with employers to make vaccination shots available at more work sites or, barring that, encourage employers to provide employees paid time off to get vaccinated at a nearby facility. Finally, the government plan would create more mobile clinics, including at special events, summer festivals, sporting events, places of worship, and "wherever we can find people gathered."[63]

Reflecting the lack of national consensus in responding to the pandemic, some experts criticized the plan as not doing enough and relying too much on persuasion rather than exploring the politically charged use of vaccine mandates.[65] At the same time, critics on the right accused the administration of overreach and showed how easy it is for well-intentioned remarks to turn into misinformation. In announcing the heightened efforts, the president said, "Now we need to go to community by community, neighborhood by neighborhood, and oftentimes, door to door—literally knocking on doors—to get help to the remaining people protected from the virus."[63] As an Associated Press fact check later noted, "A range of false information has circulated on social media around the effort. Some posts say the campaign would force vaccines on people while others suggest the Biden administration's initiative has a hidden agenda that will lead to guns or Bibles being confiscated."[64] Timed too closely with an announcement about the deployment of federal surge teams, the administration did not state clearly enough that local employees and volunteers would staff the door-to-door campaign, and critics conflated the two efforts.

Republicans made hay of the announcement. "The Biden administration wants to knock on your door to see if you're vaccinated,"[65] Ohio representative Jim Jordan (R-OH) tweeted. "What's next? Knocking on your door to see if you own a gun?"[65] During the Conservative Political Action Conference, then North Carolina representative Madison Cawthorn (R-NC) echoed claims that the door-to-door vaccine program could lead to gun confiscation, saying, "Think about the mechanisms they would have to build to be able to actually execute that massive of a thing. And then think about what those mechanisms could be used for. They could then go door to door and take your guns. They could go door to door and take your Bibles."[66] The episode provided a case study in how public health efforts to save lives could be twisted into fear mongering to win political points.

The White House, which had rarely directly engaged with critics up to that point, decided it was time to push back. White House press secretary Jen Psaki attempted some clarification at a press conference on July 9, saying, "This is grassroots volunteers, this is members of the clergy, these are volunteers who believe that people across the country, especially in low-vaccinated areas, should have accurate information, should have information about where they can get vaccinated, where they can save their own lives and their neighbors' lives and their family members' lives."[67] Criticizing the misinformation about the door-to-door efforts, White House COVID Task Force coordinator Jeff Zients said, "For those individuals, organizations that are feeding misinformation and trying to mischaracterize this type of trusted-messenger work, I believe you are doing a disservice to the country and to the doctors, the faith leaders, community leaders and others who are working to get people vaccinated, save lives and help end this pandemic."[68]

A PANDEMIC OF THE UNVACCINATED?

By mid-July 2021, cases were rising despite the heightened efforts to get more people vaccinated. On July 17, President Biden made a comment that, while accurate, may have further polarized the vaccination effort. "Look, the only pandemic we have is among the unvaccinated,"[69] the president said that day. The remark drew subsequent criticism from a range of experts who said it risked unintentionally stigmatizing the very people who needed to be persuaded. It also diverted from the focus on condemning the misinformation driving hesitancy and seeing the unvaccinated as the victims of misinformation.[70] The message was also complicated by the increasing emergence of breakthrough infections among the vaccinated that caused both cynicism and distrust among some portions of the public.

The first small step in the Biden administration's move from persuasion to mandates, or what some viewed as coercion, came on July 29, 2021, when the president directed the DoD to look into how to add COVID-19 vaccination to the list of required vaccinations for members of the military. While current military members are well aware that they are required to be up to date on at least nine vaccines upon entering basic training (and more depending on area of deployment),[71] the politicized nature of COVID created quite a kerfuffle when this announcement was made. On August 12, 2021, HHS announced plans to mandate vaccination for all staff who serve in federally operated health care and clinical research facilities. The following week, on August 18, the White House announced HHS would develop new regulations requiring nursing homes to require all employees to be fully vaccinated as a condition of participating in Medicare and Medicaid.

But the most far-reaching announcement came on September 9, 2021. In remarks at the White House, the president announced that the Department of Labor would develop an emergency rule to require all employers with 100 or more employees to ensure their workforce was fully vaccinated or showed a negative COVID-19 test at least once a week (it would also require employers with 100 or more workers to give those workers paid time off to get vaccinated).[72] He also announced executive orders requiring all executive branch federal employees and contractors to be vaccinated and reiterated that HHS was developing regulations requiring health care workers in hospitals, home health care facilities, or other medical facilities that treat Medicare and Medicaid patients to be fully vaccinated. Speaking directly to the unvaccinated, the president's remarks were punctuated by this remarkable appeal:

> We've been patient, but our patience is wearing thin. And your refusal has cost all of us. So, please, do the right thing. But just don't take it from me; listen to the voices of unvaccinated Americans who are lying in hospital beds, taking their final breaths, saying, "If only I had gotten vaccinated. If only." It's a tragedy. Please don't let it become yours.[72]

The administration's proposals set off a predictable firestorm, with conservative state officials quickly filing a slew of lawsuits to block the proposed rules. Quickly reaching the US Supreme Court, the justices issued a split decision on January 13, 2022, upholding the federal government's authority to mandate vaccine for health care workers at institutions participating in Medicare and Medicaid but blocking the employer regulation, saying the Department of Labor lacked explicit congressional authority to issue such an emergency rule.[73,74]

Despite these immense challenges, the number of COVID vaccines administered over the first year exceeded by far the number of any previous American campaign. As 2021 came to a close, the nation had administered over 500 million doses and provided protection to over 80% of all adults.[75] It was simply an unprecedented achievement and could not have happened without the dedication of tens of thousands of public health professionals and private-sector partners.

However, there remained a sizable percentage of the population that continued to either delay vaccination or outright refuse COVID vaccine. Overcoming vaccine hesitancy would become an ever-greater challenge for public health and health care leaders in the months ahead, as it seemed efforts to build vaccine confidence had hit a wall.

REFERENCES

1. Falconer R. Misinformation spurring US life expectancy "erosion," FDA chief says. *Axios*. May 7, 2022. Available at: https://www.axios.com/2022/05/08/misinformation-us-life-expectancy-drop-fda-chief. Accessed September 16, 2022.
2. McGraw M. Trump encourages Americans to get the Covid vaccine. *Politico*. March 16, 2021. Available at: https://www.politico.com/news/2021/03/16/trump-americans-covid-vaccine-476479. Accessed September 16, 2022.
3. Otterman S. "I trust science," says nurse who is first to get vaccine in US. *New York Times*. December 14, 2020. Available at: https://www.nytimes.com/2020/12/14/nyregion/us-covid-vaccine-first-sandra-lindsay.html. Accessed September 16, 2022.

4. Andrew Cuomo: Watch LIVE as the first person in New York gets vaccinated. *Periscope*. December 14, 2020. Available at: https://www.pscp.tv/w/1eaKbnZRXjqKX. Accessed September 16, 2022.

5. The COVID Tracking Project. Totals for the US. Available at: https://covidtracking.com/data/national. Accessed September 16, 2022.

6. US Government Accountability Office. COVID-19: efforts to increase vaccine availability and perspectives on initial implementation. April 2021. Available at: https://www.gao.gov/assets/gao-21-443.pdf. Accessed September 16, 2022.

7. Roubein R. Warp Speed official takes blame for overcount of Covid shot allocations. *Politico*. December 19, 2020. Available at: https://www.politico.com/news/2020/12/19/coronavirus-vaccine-overcount-warp-speed-448692. Accessed September 16, 2022.

8. Brenan M. Satisfaction with US vaccine rollout surges to 68%. Gallup. March 30, 2021. Available at: https://news.gallup.com/poll/342431/satisfaction-vaccine-rollout-surges.aspx. Accessed September 16, 2022.

9. National Archives and Records Administration. Remarks by President Trump on vaccine development. May 15, 2020. Available at: https://trumpwhitehouse.archives.gov/briefings-statements/remarks-president-trump-vaccine-development. Accessed September 16, 2022.

10. Blake A, Rieger JM. The Trump administration is delivering on a 2020 vaccine, but not at the levels the president suggested. *Washington Post*. December 10, 2020. Available at: https://www.washingtonpost.com/politics/2020/12/10/trump-administration-is-delivering-2020-vaccine-not-levels-he-suggested. Accessed September 16, 2022.

11. Mason J. Trump to meet next week with industry, government officials on COVID vaccine. *Reuters*. December 1, 2020. Available at: https://www.reuters.com/article/us-health-coronavirus-vaccines-trump/trump-to-meet-next-week-with-industry-government-officials-on-covid-vaccine-idUSKBN28B69R. Accessed September 16, 2022.

12. McArdle M. White House expects to distribute 20 million coronavirus vaccine doses by December. *National Review*. November 13, 2020. Available at: https://www.nationalreview.com/news/white-house-expects-to-distribute-20-million-coronavirus-vaccine-doses-by-december. Accessed September 16, 2022.

13. McKesson. Standing ready: a documentary short. Available at: https://www.mckesson.com/About-McKesson/COVID-19-Documentary. Accessed September 16, 2022.

14. Ibarra AB. Californians ask: where are our coronavirus vaccines? *CalMatters*. January 29, 2021. Updated September 28, 2021. Available at: https://calmatters.org/health/coronavirus/2021/01/californians-ask-where-are-our-coronavirus-vaccines. Accessed September 16, 2022.

15. Harris R. Why the COVID-19 vaccine distribution has gotten off to a slow start. *Morning Edition*. National Public Radio. January 1, 2021. Available at: https://www.npr.org/2021/01/01/952652202/why-the-covid-19-vaccine-distribution-has-gotten-off-to-a-slow-start. Accessed September 16, 2022.

16. Mackintosh E. As the world begins its vaccination push, delayed rollouts draw criticism and concern. *CNN*. January 11, 2021. Available at: https://www.cnn.com/2021/01/11/world/vaccine-rollout-delays-intl. Accessed September 16, 2022.

17. Here & Now. Governors frustrated with slow COVID-19 vaccine rollout. WBUR. January 18, 2021. Available at: https://www.wbur.org/hereandnow/2021/01/18/covid-19-vaccine-states-trump. Accessed September 16, 2022.

18. Rev. Operation Warp Speed COVID-19 press conference transcript by defense officials, January 12. January 12, 2021. Available at: https://www.rev.com/blog/transcripts/operation-warp-speed-covid-19-press-conference-transcript-by-defense-officials-january-12. Accessed September 16, 2022.

19. Leonhardt D. Britain's "one-jab" strategy. *New York Times.* March 19, 2021. Available at: https://www.nytimes.com/2021/03/19/briefing/atlanta-shootings-ncaa-mens-division-teen-vogue.html. Accessed September 16, 2022.

20. Rev. HHS briefing on Operation Warp Speed, vaccine distribution transcript December 2. December 2, 2020. Available at: https://www.rev.com/blog/transcripts/hhs-briefing-on-operation-warp-speed-vaccine-distribution-transcript-december-2. Accessed September 16, 2022.

21. Stanley-Becker I, Sun LH. Vaccine reserve was exhausted when Trump administration vowed to release it, dashing hopes of expanded access. *Washington Post.* January 15, 2021. Available at: https://www.washingtonpost.com/health/2021/01/15/trump-vaccine-reserve-used-up. Accessed September 16, 2022.

22. Centers for Disease Control and Prevention. COVID-19 vaccination program interim playbook for jurisdictions operations annex. January 2022. Available at: https://www.cdc.gov/vaccines/covid-19/covid19-vaccination-guidance.html. Accessed September 16, 2022.

23. O'Donnell C, Spalding R. Local funding crisis threatens US vaccine rollout. *Reuters.* December 31, 2020. Available at: https://www.reuters.com/article/health-coronavirus-vaccines-distribution-idINKBN29620V. Accessed September 16, 2022.

24. Esper MT. *A Sacred Oath: Memoirs of a Secretary of Defense during Extraordinary Times.* New York, NY: William Morrow, an imprint of HarperCollins Publishers; 2022.

25. Roussel A. Business as Usual: Paul Mango of Operation Warp Speed. [Transcript]. Pittsburgh Technology Council. December 21, 2020. Available at: https://www.pghtech.org/programs/BAUxPaulMangoOpWarpSpeed. Accessed September 16, 2022.

26. Cunningham PW. Operation Warp Speed chief says coronavirus vaccine distribution is "working perfectly." *Washington Post.* January 15, 2021. Available at: https://www.washingtonpost.com/politics/2021/01/15/health-202-operation-warp-speed-chief-says-coronavirus-vaccine-distribution-is-working-perfectly. Accessed September 16, 2022.

27. New York State. National Governors Association submits list of questions to Trump administration on effective implementation of COVID-19 vaccine. October 18, 2020. Available at: https://www.governor.ny.gov/news/national-governors-association-submits-list-questions-trump-administration-effective. Accessed September 16, 2022.

28. US Department of Health and Human Services. Answers to National Governors Association questions on vaccine distribution and planning. Available at: https://www.hhs.gov/sites/default/files/national-governors-association-questions-on-vaccine-distribution-planning.pdf. Accessed September 16, 2022.

29. Centers for Disease Control and Prevention. COVID-19 vaccination supplemental funding. January 2021. Available at: https://www.cdc.gov/vaccines/covid-19/downloads/vaccination-supplemental-funding.pdf. Accessed September 16, 2022.

30. Centers for Disease Control and Prevention. Covid-19 vaccination Federal Retail Pharmacy Partnership Program. July 11, 2022. Available at: https://www.cdc.gov/vaccines/covid-19/retail-pharmacy-program/index.html. Accessed September 16, 2022.

31. Mitropoulos A. One year of COVID-19 vaccines: millions inoculated, but hundreds of thousands still lost. *ABC News*. December 14, 2021. Available at: https://abcnews.go.com/US/year-covid-19-vaccines-millions-inoculated-hundreds-thousands/story?id=81629912. Accessed September 16, 2022.

32. Feuer W. President-elect Joe Biden announces Covid task force. *CNBC Health and Science*. November 7, 2020. Available at: https://www.cnbc.com/2020/11/07/president-elect-joe-biden-to-announce-covid-task-force-on-monday.html. Accessed September 16, 2022.

33. The White House. National strategy for the COVID-19 response and pandemic preparedness. January 2021. Available at: https://www.whitehouse.gov/wp-content/uploads/2021/01/National-Strategy-for-the-COVID-19-Response-and-Pandemic-Preparedness.pdf. Accessed September 16, 2022.

34. Siddiqui S, Alpert L. Biden says Trump administration's vaccine plan is falling behind. *Wall Street Journal*. December 29, 2020. Available at: https://www.wsj.com/livecoverage/covid-2020-12-29/card/84FaGV9L3fo7aerapFS2. Accessed September 16, 2022.

35. NBC News. Meet the Press—January 24, 2021. [Transcript]. January 24, 2021. Available at: https://www.nbcnews.com/meet-the-press/meet-press-january-24-2021-n1255457. Accessed September 16, 2022.

36. The White House. Remarks by President Biden on the fight to contain the COVID-19 pandemic. January 26, 2021. Available at: https://www.whitehouse.gov/briefing-room/speeches-remarks/2021/01/26/remarks-by-president-biden-on-the-fight-to-contain-the-covid-19-pandemic. Accessed September 16, 2022.

37. Whitaker B. How the United States plans to increase the pace of COVID-19 vaccinations. *60 Minutes/CBS News*. February 28, 2021. Available at: https://www.cbsnews.com/news/covid-vaccine-shots-in-arms-60-minutes-2021-02-28/?ftag=CNM-00-10aab7d&linkId=112454650. Accessed September 16, 2022.

38. The White House. Remarks by President Biden at an event commemorating the 50 millionth COVID-19 vaccine shot. February 25, 2021. Available at: https://www.whitehouse.gov/briefing-room/speeches-remarks/2021/02/25/remarks-by-president-biden-at-an-event-commemorating-the-50-millionth-covid-19-vaccine-shot. Accessed September 16, 2022.

39. Parker K. If you got a vaccine, Trump wants you to thank him. *Washington Post*. March 12, 2021. Available at: https://www.washingtonpost.com/opinions/donald-trump-wants-credit-for-the-vaccine-as-if/2021/03/12/4f40a492-836e-11eb-81db-b02f0398f49a_story.html. Accessed September 16, 2022.

40. Flaherty A, Pezenik S. "The mess we inherited": Biden leans heavily on Trump's "Warp Speed" but won't give credit. *ABC News*. March 11, 2021. Available at: https://abcnews.go.com/Politics/mess-inherited-biden-leans-heavily-trumps-warp-speed/story?id=76186823. Accessed September 16, 2022.

41. Leonard B. Slavitt: I would "tip my hat" to Trump's Operation Warp Speed. *Politico*. March 11, 2021. Available at: https://www.politico.com/news/2021/03/11/slavitt-trump-operation-warp-speed-475310. Accessed September 16, 2022.

42. Sherman A. Trump vaccine plan left logistics to states, but it did exist. *Politifact*. January 27, 2021. Available at: https://www.politifact.com/factchecks/2021/jan/27/ron-klain/trump-vaccine-plan-left-logistics-states-it-did-ex. Accessed September 16, 2022.

43. US Department of Health and Human Services. Barda's first 15 years. February 1, 2022. Available at: https://www.medicalcountermeasures.gov/stories/barda15. September 16, 2022.

44. US Government Accountability Office. COVID-19: HHS and DOD transitioned vaccine responsibilities to HHS, but need to address outstanding issues. January 2022. Available at: https://www.gao.gov/assets/gao-22-104453.pdf. Accessed September 16, 2022.

45. US Government Accountability Office. COVID-19 HHS agencies' planned reviews of vaccine distribution and communication efforts should include stakeholder perspectives. November 4, 2021. Available at: https://www.gao.gov/products/gao-22-104457. Accessed September 16, 2022.

46. Stanley-Becker I. FEMA would operate up to 100 federally run mass vaccination sites under Biden plan. *Washington Post*. January 22, 2021. Available at: https://www.washingtonpost .com/health/2021/01/22/biden-vaccine-mass-sites. Accessed September 16, 2022.

47. Federal Emergency Management Agency. FEMA COVID-19 update. Release number HQ-21-107. May 14, 2021. Available at: https://www.fema.gov/press-release/20210514/fema-covid-19-update. Accessed September 16, 2022.

48. Health Resources and Services Administration. Ensuring equity in COVID-19 vaccine distribution. Available at: https://www.hrsa.gov/coronavirus/health-center-program. Accessed September 16, 2022.

49. Health Resources and Services Administration. Health center COVID-19 vaccinations among racial and ethnic minority patients. Available at: https://data.hrsa.gov/topics/health-centers/covid-vaccination. Accessed September 16, 2022.

50. Centers for Disease Control and Prevention. Joint CDC and FDA statement on Johnson & Johnson COVID-19 vaccine. April 13, 2021. Available at: https://www.cdc.gov/media/releases/2021/s0413-JJ-vaccine.html. Accessed September 16, 2022.

51. Oliver SE, Wallace M, See I, et al. Use of the Janssen (Johnson & Johnson) COVID-19 vaccine: updated interim recommendations from the Advisory Committee on Immunization Practices—United States, December 2021. *MMWR Morbidity and Mortality Weekly Report*. 2022;71(3):90–95. doi:10.15585/mmwr.mm7103a4.

52. Berg S. What doctors wish patients knew about the Johnson & Johnson vaccine. American Medical Association. November 4, 2021. Available at: https://www.ama-assn.org/delivering-care/public-health/what-doctors-wish-patients-knew-about-johnson-johnson-vaccine. Accessed September 16, 2022.

53. The White House. Remarks by President Biden on the administration's COVID-19 vaccination efforts. March 2, 2021. Available at: https://www.whitehouse.gov/briefing-room/speeches-remarks/2021/03/02/remarks-by-president-biden-on-the-administrations-covid-19-vaccination-efforts. Accessed September 16, 2022.

54. The White House. Fact sheet: President Biden announces 90% of the adult US population will be eligible for vaccination and 90% will have a vaccination site within 5 miles of home by April 19. March 29, 2021. Available at: https://www.whitehouse.gov/briefing-room/statements-releases/2021/03/29/fact-sheet-president-biden-announces-90-of-the-adult-u-s-population-will-be-eligible-for-vaccination-and-90-will-have-a-vaccination-site-within-5-miles-of-home-by-april-19. Accessed September 16, 2022.

55. The White House. Fact sheet: President Biden to announce goal to administer at least one vaccine shot to 70% of the US adult population by July 4th. May 4, 2021. Available at:

https://www.whitehouse.gov/briefing-room/statements-releases/2021/05/04/fact-sheet-president-biden-to-announce-goal-to-administer-at-least-one-vaccine-shot-to-70-of-the-u-s-adult-population-by-july-4th. Accessed September 16, 2022.

56. The White House. National month of action for COVID-19 vaccinations. June 3, 2021. Available at: https://www.whitehouse.gov/national-month-of-action. Accessed September 16, 2022.

57. Roy M. Delta variant already dominant in US, CDC estimates show. *Reuters*. July 7, 2021. Available at: https://www.reuters.com/world/us/delta-variant-already-dominant-us-cdc-estimates-show-2021-07-07. Accessed September 16, 2022.

58. Hamel L, Kearney A, Kirzinger A, Lopes L, Munana C, Brodie M. KFF Health Tracking Poll—September 2020: top issues in 2020 election, the role of misinformation, and views on a potential coronavirus vaccine. KFF. September 10, 2020. Available at: https://www.kff.org/coronavirus-covid-19/report/kff-health-tracking-poll-september-2020. Accessed September 16, 2022.

59. Kirzinger A, Kearney A, Hamel L, Brodie M. KFF COVID-19 Vaccine Monitor: The increasing importance of partisanship in predicting COVID-19 vaccination status. KFF. November 16, 2021. Available at: https://www.kff.org/coronavirus-covid-19/poll-finding/importance-of-partisanship-predicting-vaccination-status. Accessed September 16, 2022.

60. Jones JM. Americans' optimism about covid-19 dashed as cases surge. Gallup. August 2, 2021. Available at: https://news.gallup.com/poll/353003/americans-optimism-covid-dashed-cases-surge.aspx. Accessed September 16, 2022.

61. McEvoy J. 32 states didn't hit Biden's July 4 vaccine goal—these were the furthest from it. *Forbes*. July 4, 2021. Available at: https://www.forbes.com/sites/jemimamcevoy/2021/07/04/32-states-didnt-hit-bidens-july-4-vaccine-goal-these-were-the-furthest-from-it. Accessed September 16, 2022.

62. The White House. Remarks by President Biden on the COVID-19 response and the vaccination program. July 6, 2021. Available at: https://www.whitehouse.gov/briefing-room/speeches-remarks/2021/07/06/remarks-by-president-biden-on-the-covid-19-response-and-the-vaccination-program-6. Accessed September 16, 2022.

63. Shear M, Weiland N. Biden calls for door-to-door vaccine push; experts say more is needed. *New York Times*. July 6, 2021. Available at: https://www.nytimes.com/2021/07/06/us/politics/biden-vaccines.html. Accessed September 16, 2022.

64. The Associated Press. Online reports mislead on vaccination door-knocking efforts. *AP News*. July 14, 2021. Available at: https://apnews.com/article/fact-checking-680185772094. Accessed September 16, 2022.

65. Jordan RJ (@Jim_Jordan). The Biden administration wants to knock on your door to see if you're vaccinated. what's next? knocking on your door to see if you own a gun? Twitter. Posted July 8, 2021. Available at: https://twitter.com/jim_jordan/status/1413120222991634434?lang=en. Accessed September 16, 2022.

66. Ellington AJ. Madison Cawthorn says door-to-door vaccines could lead to taking of guns, Bibles. *Newsweek*. July 9, 2021. Available at: https://www.newsweek.com/madison-cawthorn-says-door-door-vaccines-could-lead-taking-guns-bibles-1608503. Accessed September 16, 2022.

67. The White House. Press briefing by Press Secretary Jen Psaki, July 9, 2021. July 9, 2021. Available at: https://www.whitehouse.gov/briefing-room/press-briefings/2021/07/09/press-briefing-by-press-secretary-jen-psaki-july-9-2021. Accessed September 16, 2022.

68. Miller Z. White House calling out critics of door-to-door vaccine push. *AP News*. July 10, 2021. Available at: https://apnews.com/article/joe-biden-health-government-and-politics-coronavirus-pandemic-michael-brown-c5c9260bc083e7e9cc0e415caa43879f. Accessed September 14, 2022.

69. Miller Z. Biden grappling with "pandemic of the unvaccinated." *AP News*. July 17, 2021. Available at: https://apnews.com/article/joe-biden-health-government-and-politics-pandemics-coronavirus-pandemic-8318e3f406278f3ebf09871128cc91de. Accessed September 16, 2022.

70. Alonso-Zaldivar R. Questioning a catchphrase: "pandemic of the unvaccinated." *AP News*. September 1, 2021. Available at: https://apnews.com/article/health-pandemics-coronavirus-pandemic-9845c7257300ff6546c20489e642a1ea. Accessed September 16, 2022.

71. Departments of the Army, the Navy, the Air Force, and the Coast Guard Headquarters. Immunizations and Chemoprophylaxis for the Prevention of Infectious Diseases. Army Regulation 40–562. October 7, 2013. Available at: https://media.defense.gov/2017/Mar/16/2001717444/-1/-1/0/CIM_6230_4G.pdf. Accessed September 16, 2022.

72. The White House. Remarks by President Biden on fighting the COVID-19 pandemic. September 9, 2021. Available at: https://www.whitehouse.gov/briefing-room/speeches-remarks/2021/09/09/remarks-by-president-biden-on-fighting-the-covid-19-pandemic-3. Accessed September 16, 2022.

73. Barnes R. Supreme Court blocks Biden's workplace vaccine rules, allows requirement for health-care workers. *Washington Post*. January 13, 2022. Available at: https://www.washingtonpost.com/politics/courts_law/supreme-court-biden-vaccine-rules/2022/01/13/2e6e4b9e-749e-11ec-bc13-18891499c514_story.html. Accessed September 16, 2022.

74. *National Federation of Independent Business, et al., Applicants v. Department of Labor, Occupational Safety and Health Administration, et al.* 595 US (2022). Updated January 13, 2022. Available at: https://www.supremecourt.gov/opinions/21pdf/21a244_hgci.pdf. Accessed September 16, 2022.

75. Centers for Disease Control and Prevention. CDC COVID data tracker. Available at: https://covid.cdc.gov/covid-data-tracker/#vaccinations_vacc-people-additional-dose-totalpop. Accessed September 16, 2022.

Hitting the Wall

*We should not be here, y'all. This is not necessary . . . Too many people are getting informa-
tion from wrong sources . . . These Facebook conspiratorial lists are going to spread and
run, and have no accountability for the people who are dying, and we're here, picking up
the mess.[1]*

–Dr. Thomas Dobbs, Mississippi state health officer, April 13, 2021, at press event
on opening of federal emergency field hospital in a hospital parking garage
to treat overflow COVID patients at a Mississippi hospital

*I've just been conditioned not to trust . . . If we got to a place where the government says,
"OK, now it's time to take a vaccine," then I'm definitely going to be skeptical of their
intentions.[2]*

–Rahmell Peebles, Black New York City resident, interviewed
April 5, 2020, by the Associated Press

After months of shutdowns, millions of infections, and an estimated 385,000 lives lost to
COVID in 2020 in the United States, public health professionals welcomed the news of
successful vaccine trials in November and December 2020.[3] Early demand for the vaccine was high, with media reports of people eagerly waiting in line to get their shot.[4] In a
story critical of the state's early web-based vaccine appointment system rollout in January
2021, CNN aired scenes of Florida seniors lined up on sidewalks waiting overnight to get
their COVID vaccine.[5] Reports of celebrities and elites eager to skip their places in line
and buy COVID vaccines from exclusive concierge physicians or clinics were also an
occurrence in the first weeks of the rollout.[6,7] Others reported driving hours to get a vaccine in another state where a vaccination appointment was available or waiting up late at
night to refresh appointment booking websites when new vaccination appointments
were added.

Demand for vaccines certainly outpaced supply in the early weeks and months of the
US vaccination campaign: vaccine allocation and ordering details and dealing with
shortages were a constant item on almost daily state health official calls with the Centers
for Disease Control and Prevention (CDC), Department of Health and Human Services
(HHS), and White House staff.

But many Americans also had questions and concerns about the safety of these new
vaccines. Fall 2020 data on intent to be vaccinated were a preview of the hesitancy some
Americans felt about getting their shot. When asked if a free vaccine was available before

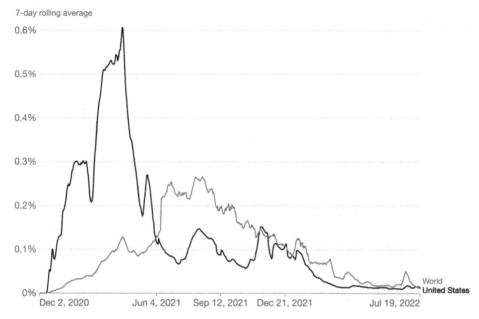

Source: Our World in Data.[10] Reprinted via open access under CC BY 4.0 license (https://creativecommons.org/licenses/by/4.0).

Figure 7-1. Daily Share of Population Receiving a First COVID-19 Dose

the election, just 4 in 10 adults (42%) said they would want to get vaccinated.[8] In the early days of the rollout, not all health care workers wanted to, nor were all seniors as enthusiastic as those waiting in line in Florida. States soon moved to other priority groups as demand among the first groups softened, opening eligibility to people age 50 or over and then, at President Biden's request, to all eligible adults by May 1, 2021.[9]

COVID vaccine uptake in the United States peaked in April 2021, with a downward trend in the months thereafter (see Figure 7-1).[10] Demand ebbed and flowed in the summer and fall of 2021, but by the end of 2021, it had stagnated: we had hit a wall.

ANTICIPATING HESITANCY

Public health officials anticipated a substantial degree of COVID vaccine hesitancy because of rising anti-vaccination activism prior to COVID. This problem started well before COVID arrived on our doorstep and went beyond America's borders: in 2019, the World Health Organization included vaccine hesitancy as one of its top 10 global health threats.[11] Health officers dealt with sporadic outbreaks of vaccine-preventable childhood diseases among the unvaccinated such as pertussis and measles in the years before COVID, although these were isolated regional outbreaks and usually specific to a particular community.

While anticipating some degree of vaccine hesitancy in the COVID vaccination campaign, many health officials were surprised by the extent of hesitancy in so many groups, including some health care workers and nursing home staff.[12,13] Prevalent misinformation and disinformation about the vaccine's development over multiple social media platforms and the politicization of the COVID vaccine by both Republicans and Democrats, in conjunction with many questions about the broad use of new "mRNA" vaccine technology, helped spur these concerns. Conspiracy theorists were eager to suggest that the vaccine would allow the government to track individuals by using microchips, "quantum dots," or other invasive tracking-device technology supposedly developed by Bill Gates, for example.[14,15]

In a December 12, 2021, oral interview with North Dakota's immunization program manager Molly Howell, MPH, she told us:

> And anticipating hesitancy[,] it felt like it just came all at once. I'm not naïve, I knew there would be some, but it felt just like hitting a wall . . . I think it's a different type of hesitancy than we've ever seen before. I think its political and we have to acknowledge that, and we're going to have to change. I think we are making some inroads. We're really transparent with our data where people can see the differences in vaccinated versus unvaccinated rates themselves. And we are relying on physicians throughout the state to more be the spokespeople for vaccine than the department. It's just going to be small incremental steps.

Politicians were eager to use the concerns about the speed of vaccine development as talking points in election campaigning even before a vaccine was approved for use in the United States: President Trump wanted to take credit for its development in his reelection bid, while the Biden–Harris campaign raised questions about political interference in the regulatory approval and cited a lack of confidence in Trump's vaccine rollout plan in theirs.[16] In a virtual plenary session at a journalism conference on August 6, 2020, then candidate Biden said:

> The way he [Trump] talks about the vaccine is not particularly rational. He's talking about it being ready, he's going to talk about moving it quicker than the scientists think it should be moved . . . People don't believe that he's telling the truth, therefore they're not at all certain they're going to take the vaccine. And one more thing: If and when the vaccine comes, it's not likely to go through all the tests that need to be done, and the trials that are needed to be done.[17]

Indeed, as the vaccine distribution launched in December 2020, more than one-third of all Americans (39%) told pollsters that they would "wait and see" how the vaccine is working for others before getting vaccinated themselves.[18] Dr. Tom Frieden noted in our June 10, 2022, oral interview with him that the speed of development created what he called a rational hesitation. "It *was* pretty fast that there were remarkably effective vaccines available," he told us, "and that has led to some of the questions because people say, you know, it can't be right, [so] when you think of the folks who've been hesitant, it's a rational hesitation." Fortunately, however, as the extraordinary safety record of the vaccines became clear after millions of injections worldwide, the number of Americans taking the wait-and-see approach declined quickly to 31% in January and 22% by February 2021.[18]

By the summer of 2021, hesitancy took an even more political bent as trust in the authorities recommending vaccination declined with an ever-increasing onslaught of vaccine misinformation and disinformation and growing anti-public health sentiment. Trust is built through relationships, and the science of health promotion is fundamentally based on how health care and public health workers can establish trusting relationships that encourage healthy behaviors in their patients over time. In our December 13, 2021, oral interview with Paul Mango, MBA, he shared with us his regret that Operation Warp Speed did not have a single behavioral health scientist on its team, stating:

> There were a bunch of virologists and epidemiologists who were "the experts." We didn't have a single behavioral scientist on the team. And if you think about COVID in retrospect its all about behavior modification—everything, whether travel, social distancing, wear a mask, get vaccinated. All about behavior modification. We didn't have a single behavioral scientist on the team. I think we should have. It is a science . . . there are tried-and-true techniques to change behavior and we didn't adhere to that.

Behavioral health experts could have helped anticipate many of the barriers to vaccine confidence and acceptance and supported efforts to address them early on. This deficiency was another casualty of Operation Warp Speed leadership's lack of trust in the CDC, which has at least 300 behavioral scientists among its ranks.[19]

While these professionals were engaged in vaccine confidence-building activities after the vaccine launch, it is an open question if the Trump team could have made a difference by getting out front of the clear signs that hesitancy would become an issue before the initial wave of demand tapered off. The bottom line is that as of fall 2020, just months before vaccines would be rolled out across the nation, there was neither a well-funded nor a comprehensive national plan to address vaccine hesitancy systematically across the country by using core principles of health behavior to help motivate individuals to get vaccinated. In addition, no clear plan was in place to educate Americans on the rigorous safety and effectiveness review process. This included missed opportunities highlighting the tens of thousands of individuals who had participated in vaccine clinical trials and numerous independent reviews of the data submitted by manufacturers to assure safety.

CHANGING GOAL POSTS

Even as they were rolling out new vaccines in December 2020, it was apparent to most state and local health officials that significant national leadership and additional federal resources would be needed to help support vaccine confidence efforts and address rapidly growing misinformation and disinformation about the vaccine. In April 2021, HHS and the Biden White House launched their We Can Do This campaign to share information about vaccine confidence through celebrity influencers such as Mark Cuban, Ryan Seacrest, Ana Navarro, NASCAR drivers, and WNBA and NBA players, among other spokespersons.[20] The HHS COVID-19 Community Corps enrolled thousands of individuals and organizations to share vaccine confidence messages at the local level and with state and national constituents.[21] This effort featured creative materials such as the Veterans Coalition for Vaccination's riff on the famous World War II Rosie the Riveter poster and "We Can Do This" slogan with updated images and captions such as "Armward Toward Victory," "Roll-Up Your Sleeve and Crush the Virus," and "Better Times Are Within Arm's Reach."[22] By May 2021, several states sponsored lotteries and incentive programs to promote vaccination: it was clear all options were on the table to promote COVID vaccination.[23]

As described in Chapter 5, President Biden set a goal in May 2021 of 70% of all eligible Americans getting at least one dose of vaccine by July 4, 2021.[24] The goal was reached, sort of, with 70% of all Americans over age 27 being vaccinated just a few days after. In remarks from the White House, the president stated:

> Today, after receiving a briefing from my entire COVID-19 team, I'm proud to announce that we're getting even closer, because of our wartime effort, to administer thr—to administer 300 million shots in arms in just 150 days. More than 182 million Americans have received at least one shot, including nearly 90 percent of seniors and 70 percent of adults over the age of 27. By the end of this week, we'll have reached the mark of 160 million fully vaccinated Americans. And that's a goal I set in March that I'm thrilled we're going to hit just a few days after July the Fourth. So, we will have 160 million fully vaccinated Americans—up from roughly 3 million when we took office five months ago . . . This is one of the greatest achievements in American history, and you, the American people, made it happen . . . Now we need to go to community by community, neighborhood by neighborhood, and oftentimes, door to door—literally knocking on doors—to get help to the remaining people protected from the virus.[25]

To achieve this goal, the nation's federal, state, and local health officials had declared an all-out war on vaccine hesitancy. With support from the Biden administration and Congress, health departments initially focused on access and convenience, using mobile vans to provide vaccination clinics in hard-to-reach areas, staffing drive-in vaccine clinics in sports stadiums and mall parking lots, and funding community-based organizations and local health authorities. But despite millions of dollars and many state and local efforts to create innovative public relations materials and expand available locations to be vaccinated, vaccine demand still plateaued. It was clear that a sizable percentage of the US population had decided to wait longer or forgo entirely their shot at a COVID vaccine.

Both vaccine hesitancy and vaccine refusal are bewildering to many of us. The development of vaccines has been hailed as one of the greatest public health achievements in the 21st century because of their impact on reducing morbidity and mortality. Because vaccines are lifesaving and cost effective, public health and health care professionals have been encouraging child and adult vaccination for vaccine-preventable diseases for decades. UNICEF, the United Nations International Children's Emergency Fund, attributes two to three million children's lives saved annually as a result of childhood vaccination programs worldwide, with the number of children paralyzed by polio falling 99% since 1988.[26]

A 2015 review of the economic value of vaccines overall found that for every dollar the United States spends on vaccinations, $3 is saved in direct health care costs and $10 in indirect social costs, including missed days of work: spending $1 to save $13 is quite a deal.[27] The CDC estimates the vaccination of children born between 1994 and 2018 has saved the United States nearly $406 billion in medical costs that would have otherwise been associated with vaccine-preventable diseases. Vaccines are not just about preventing childhood diseases, however.[28] The CDC also estimates that as a nation we spend $27 billion a year on treating vaccine-preventable diseases in Americans over age 50, including influenza, pneumococcal disease, and shingles.[28]

In the months leading up to COVID vaccine's authorization and thereafter, many health officials, the media, and members of the public speculated about the percentage of the public that would need to be vaccinated to confer immunity among the US population. Given the continued spread of illness in July 2021, it was clear that 70% was not enough, but it was also unclear what percentage would be enough to reach herd immunity. *Herd immunity* is an epidemiological term used to describe the protection a community has against an infectious disease when a significant percentage of the population is no longer susceptible to a disease either through vaccination or through natural infection.[29] This percentage varies widely depending on the disease and its infectiousness: the more infectious the disease, the more people that need to become immune to snuff it out and keep it from spreading to those who are not immune. Measles, for example, is a highly contagious disease that requires 95% of the population to be immune to stop transmission.[30]

Estimates of the necessary rate of herd immunity for COVID varied as more was learned about the virus and its transmissibility, starting with an initial estimate of 60% to 70% in the early months of the pandemic.[31,32] Later, in late summer and fall 2021, experts such as Dr. Anthony Fauci considered a rate of 90% or higher auspicous.[33] A continuously moving target, this ever-changing estimate raised public frustration and perhaps contributed to undermining trust in public health authorities.

In our February 25, 2022, oral interview with Kelly Moore, MD, MPH, of *immunize .org*, she shared her view on how the variant's changing transmission rates and resulting changing estimates of herd immunity created such a vexing challenge:

Once your reproductive number is in the range of measles, you have to have at least 95% of people immune to achieve herd immunity. So the public does not understand that the goal posts move when the R-naught (R_0) moves, and they just got mad that the goal posts were moving and not realizing the virus is the thing moving the goal posts, not us. So from a communications standpoint, it was problematic because people didn't understand where that 70% number came from. And the fact that it only works, if you keep [transmissibility] down to as low as original COVID was, but Delta moved the goal post.

Hesitancy took its toll on the public health professionals and health care providers who did support vaccination. Many were harassed by individuals opposed to vaccination (anti-vaxxers) for their efforts to promote and mandate vaccines, along with other public health mitigation efforts such as masking and social distancing.[34,35,36] Public health officials we interviewed described the difficulty in personally reconciling the tragedy of having a safe, effective, and free COVID vaccine and yet seeing hundreds of thousands of mostly unvaccinated people dying from COVID-related illness after the vaccine became available in practically every community in America.

Claire Hannan, MPH, told us in our March 17, 2022, oral interview how this unfolding situation concerned the public health community: "I think that's when we really started worrying about the mental health of our immunization program managers because that's really when they were staying up all night and putting in orders, and finding more nurses, and looking at what other states were doing to address the problems they were having, and trying all these new things, and it doesn't seem to help. That's where you really start to realize that this is tragic. These people are not taking the vaccine. That probably is the hardest thing."

Social scientists and public health researchers have shown for years that vaccine confidence, hesitancy, and refusal are rooted in deeply held beliefs and opinions, and decisions to get vaccinated are made in a social and political context. Decisions to be vaccinated, or to delay or refuse vaccination, do not always appear to be rational but make sense when you dig below the surface of what appears to some to be an irrational choice. The decision to be vaccinated depends on an individual's life experience, social network, and beliefs and truths that may appear irrational to others. Understanding these factors in the case of COVID is important to describing why we hit a proverbial vaccine wall and determining what to do about it in the future.

In February 2022, former president Bill Clinton made the case for making a better argument when he interviewed rock musician Jason Isbell for Clinton's podcast entitled *Why Am I Telling You This?* Isbell, in addition to being a brilliant songwriter and performer, had gained notoriety as a southern rocker who would perform only at venues that required audience members to be vaccinated. Clinton related to Isbell the difficulty he was having trying to persuade people to take the vaccine, saying, "But the death rate is still 13 to 16 times higher for people who aren't vaccinated than for people who are.

And I don't understand why that's not enough . . . And I wish I could make the argument better than I apparently have, because there's still a lot of people holding out out there."[37] Isbell responded, "Yeah, there are." He then offered an insightful endorsement for the need for humility in the face of such frustration, saying, "And I like the way you say that, that you wish you could make the argument better, rather than saying, 'I wish these bone-heads would understand what I'm saying.'"

Critical to addressing hesitancy is to make a better argument for vaccines than against, not to assume that the hesitant are "boneheads" or just being stubborn. But the better argument does not mean arguing solely with data and facts. Since hesitancy can come from deeply held beliefs, not a lack of information, understanding those beliefs is critical. Anti-vaccination viewpoints are often rooted in libertarian ideology, beliefs in the need for limited or "small" government, and the primacy of individual choice as opposed to collective good. They are also entrenched in myths and bad science that have been exploited by anti-vaccination advocates for years to support their position.

ORIGINS OF THE MODERN ANTI-VAXX SENTIMENT

While the modern era of vaccines is generally attributed to the development of a polio vaccine in the 1950s, scientists had been working on vaccines for over 200 years since Edward Jenner's discovery of a smallpox inoculation in 1796 and Louis Pasteur's develop-ment of the first attenuated vaccines against rabies and cholera in the 1880s. Along with these lifesaving advances, there has always been resistance and pushback. In their aptly titled article on the history of anti-vaccination sentiment "The Anti-vaccination Movement: A Regression in Modern Medicine,"[38] Hussain and colleagues summarize over 200 years of opposition to vaccination, which grew in tandem with new developments in science and medicine. Their analysis, as well as the work of others, including vaccine champion Dr. Peter Hotez, supports three common anti-vaccination themes over the course of vac-cine history: opposition on religious grounds and beliefs that vaccines oppose God's will or violate religious doctrine; opposition to allopathic medicine in favor of natural treatments and remedies used by traditional or complementary medicine, including homeopathic, osteopathic, chiropractic, or naturopathic healing; and opposition to local, state, or national government mandates, such as mandatory vaccination for school entry, that are viewed as interfering with individual or parental rights and freedoms.

When mandatory childhood vaccination for smallpox became law in the 1850s in England and penalties were established for failing to inoculate one's children, pushback and protest came from those who decried the perceived violation of their personal lib-erties and their right to decide what happens to their children's bodies. Rallies against mandatory vaccination were reported and resulted in the eventual removal of penalties for noncompliance and the creation of a conscientious objector clause that allowed for exemptions from vaccination.[39]

In 2022, the US National Conference of State Legislatures reported that all 50 states have legislation requiring immunization for school entry, but 44 states grant religious exemptions, and 15 states have laws that allow for philosophical exemptions based on parents' beliefs that their children do not need to be or should not be vaccinated.[40] Recent large measles outbreaks in the US West Coast states,[41,42] in New York,[43] and in Minnesota[44,45] have spurred some state public health efforts to remove philosophical exemptions, but success in doing so has been mixed.

Anti-vaccination sentiment came to the United States soon after the British protests around smallpox inoculation in the 1850s. In 1902, Henning Jacobson, a resident of Cambridge, Massachusetts, sued the city's board of health, which had mandated small-pox vaccination following an outbreak in the city.[46] Jacobson argued that the Massachusetts law's financial penalty (a hefty $5 at the time) or imprisonment was an "unreasonable, arbitrary, and oppressive"[47] violation of his right to choose to be vaccinated or not, and, in his view, a violation of his Fourteenth Amendment right to due process under the US Constitution. In a 7:2 decision,[48] the US Supreme Court disagreed and upheld the Massachusetts law, with Justice John Marshall Harlan writing:

> In every well-ordered society charged with the duty of conserving the safety of its members the rights of the individual in respect of his liberty may at times, under the pressure of great dangers, be subjected to such restraint, to be enforced by reasonable regulations, as the safety of the general public may demand.[49]

The Jacobson case has been the legal basis for a great deal of state public health authority, including emergency actions to protect the public's health, explicitly laying out the need for states to protect members of a society under certain circumstances even if that means (reasonably) restraining individual liberties as a result.

While there have been questions about vaccine safety throughout the 1900s, the positive safety profile and success of subsequent modern vaccines, such as the polio vaccine in the 1950s and influenza vaccination in the 1980s, generated considerable "full-throated" public support for vaccines overall.[50] Despite this support, a minority of individuals over time have had concerns about the impact of childhood vaccines on children's neurodevelopment and the use of preservatives in vaccines, such as thimerosal or adjuvants such as aluminum, as well as the schedule of vaccine administration and timing of doses for infants and young children. In 1998, however, a single research article significantly changed public perceptions of vaccine safety. Now withdrawn and discredited, the case report published in the respected British medical journal *The Lancet* in February 1998 generated immense controversy and concern about the safety of vaccines and an alleged link to developmental disabilities.[51] It is the event many historians point to as the start of the modern anti-vaxx movement.

The case report, authored by Dr. Andrew Wakefield and colleagues, reported on a group of 12 children treated in a London area hospital who had received the measles-mumps-rubella (MMR) vaccine. Within 14 days, 8 of the 12 families reported that their children began to develop signs and symptoms of the neurological and developmental disorder autism. The same children also exhibited symptoms of a novel form of inflammatory bowel disease, which Wakefield and colleagues attributed to viral replication in the colon as a result of the MMR vaccination.[50,52] The publication of Wakefield's study jolted concerned parents, scientists, and public health officials worldwide: could this in fact be true? The report's findings shook the foundations of vaccine confidence worldwide.

Fortunately for the future of scientific integrity, and unfortunately for Wakefield and his colleagues, the study was critically reviewed post-publication and substantial evidence emerged to discredit the study's methods and findings. Medical reviewers and investigators found the research was scientifically flawed and in some cases the data were either made up or misinterpreted by the researchers. The paper was formally retracted by *The Lancet* in 2010 and Wakefield's findings have never been replicated in additional studies, despite further research by Wakefield himself as well as other scientists. Wakefield resigned his academic position in Britain in 2001 and moved to the United States, where he became a prominent anti-vaccine influencer. In 2016, he produced the anti-vaccine movie *Vaxxed: From Cover-Up to Catastrophe*, and he continues to lead anti-vaxx activities today, pushing the spurious belief in a link between vaccination and developmental disorders.

There is no scientific evidence for a link between vaccines and autism, though the enduring legacy of the study is still felt today and has generated considerable vaccine hesitancy worldwide. With the publication of Wakefield's report, the genie was out of the bottle. Much of the decline in trust in vaccines, and by extension government, media, and science, can be traced to the concerns generated by this false report. The idea that vaccines cause autism and that research supporting the claim was in an internationally renowned medical journal spread rapidly. Variations on the vaccination-causes-autism theme include other unproven beliefs and myths, among them that the preservatives in vaccines cause autism (also discredited) or that the timing of multiple vaccines administered to a child overwhelms a child's immune system and causes developmental issues.

The Wakefield study caused such an uproar that the CDC asked the independent Institute of Medicine to review all published and unpublished research on the potential link. The institute released its report in 2004, which declared unequivocally, "The committee concludes that the body of epidemiological evidence favors rejection of a causal relationship between the MMR vaccine and autism."[53(p1)]

Nevertheless, anti-vaccination activists continue to push the Wakefield study's findings though discredited and retracted. In 2014, several years before being elected president, vaccine detractor Donald Trump tweeted the common falsehood, stating: "Healthy young child goes to doctor, gets pumped with massive shot of many vaccines, doesn't feel good and changes—AUTISM. Many such cases!"[54] Once elected, Donald Trump became the first vaccine skeptic to become president of the United States, a note-worthy irony, given his administration's role in advancing Operation Warp Speed.

THE RISE IN VACCINE HESITANCY AND REFUSAL

Several experts have surmised that the very success of vaccinations may be contributing to weakening support for them. As fewer people experience the morbidity and mortality caused by vaccine-preventable diseases, people may be less likely to believe that vaccines are necessary and therefore may choose not to get vaccinated. In 2008 and 2018, Research!America and the American Society for Microbiology conducted surveys in which researchers asked Americans, "Thinking about the common vaccines available today such as polio, tetanus, measles, and flu, how important do you believe vaccines are to the health of our society today?"[55] In 2008, 80% of respondents believed that vaccines were very important and 17% believed they were somewhat important. In 2018, 70% believed they were very important and 22% believed they were somewhat important. In the same surveys, researchers asked, "Do you believe you have personally benefited from the development of vaccines over the last 50 years?" In 2008, 75% said they strongly believed and 15% somewhat believed they had. In 2018, 59% said they strongly believed and 28% somewhat believed they had.

As a result of rising vaccine hesitancy and refusal, public health officials have begun to see the reemergence of vaccine-preventable diseases such as measles and pertussis. Research has demonstrated that these increases are in part a result of the reduction in vaccination rates and vaccine hesitancy among parents of school-age children. Among adults, polio is exceptionally rare in high-resource countries but may be making another debut. In May 2022, polio was detected in the United Kingdom for the first time since 1984, pushing London's health authorities to make polio boosters available to one million children in the city.[56] An unvaccinated young adult in Rockland County, New York, tested positive for polio in July 2022, sparking fears of further spread at a time when New York's health departments were already spread thin in responding to COVID and monkeypox.[57,58]

At a March 2019 US Senate Committee on Health, Education, Labor, and Pensions Committee hearing, "Vaccines Save Lives: What's Driving Preventable Disease Outbreaks?" Washington State secretary of health Dr. John Weisman stated:

> Due to the success of vaccines, fewer people have witnessed the complications and severity of vaccine preventable diseases. Unfortunately, this means that some parents may believe that vaccination is no longer necessary or that the minor or rarely severe complications from vaccines are somehow worse than getting the disease . . . In communities across Washington State and our nation, there are pockets of children who are not fully vaccinated or not vaccinated at all. This puts them at risk to contract measles and unintentionally

Table 7-1. Common Reasons for Vaccine Hesitancy and Acceptance

Common Reasons for Vaccine Hesitancy	Common Reasons for Vaccine Acceptance
• Fear of adverse effects/side effects • Concerns about vaccine safety • Mistrust or distrust of vaccine providers/ manufacturers • Low perceived risk of contracting illness • Low perceived severity of illness if infected • Belief in homeopathic/alternative medicine • Lack of information about the vaccine • Difficulty in obtaining the vaccine/access • Others will be vaccinated, so unnecessary • Experiences of racism/discrimination in health care settings	• Advice from health care provider/health care professional • Encouraged by family members, friends, colleagues • Self-protection from illness, decreased risk of illness • Belief in the overall benefits of vaccines • Social norms/expectations • Mandates for employment, for travel, for school entry, etc.

Source: Yaqub O, Castle-Clarke S, Sevdalis N, Chataway J.[60] Adapted via open access under CC BY 3.0 license (https://creativecommons.org/licenses/by/3.0).

spread it to others, especially since one is infectious with measles four days before the rash develops. It is absolutely paramount that public health and healthcare professionals across the nation join together to share the science about the safety and efficacy of vaccines with the public . . . The health concerns that parents have over the risks of vaccination must be addressed with compassion, care, and evidence-based practice.[59]

Public health and health care professionals use the term *vaccine hesitancy* to capture a continuum of reasons why parents may not vaccinate their children or adults may choose not to be vaccinated themselves. Table 7-1 summarizes some of the common reasons for hesitancy, as well as some of the reasons for vaccine acceptance.

Vaccine hesitancy is not the same as refusal. Hesitancy refers to an individual being potentially open to the possibility of being vaccinated but with questions, concerns, or the desire for more information before making that choice. Vaccine refusal refers to denying or avoiding vaccination completely for many of the reasons described earlier: religious opposition, beliefs in alternative treatments or natural remedies, and the belief that government should not compel citizens to get vaccinated. Most health officials agree that changing the minds of vaccine refusers is highly unlikely. Rather than address vaccine refusal or engage in debates with vaccine deniers, it is far more beneficial to address vaccine hesitancy by promoting vaccine confidence.

VACCINE HESITANCY: CONVENIENCE, COMPLACENCY, AND CONFIDENCE

The World Health Organization's inclusion of vaccine hesitancy as one of the 10 top global health threats was a clear indication that mounting anti-vaccination sentiment worldwide was putting populations at risk of experiencing outbreaks of many different vaccine-preventable diseases. The World Health Organization definition emphasizes three core contributors to hesitancy: convenience, complacency, and confidence.[61]

Complacency is related to the perceived risk one attributes to getting the disease a vaccine is meant to prevent. Convenience refers to how easy, or how difficult, it is to get the vaccine both in terms of location as well as affordability. Confidence relates to an individual's trust in the organizations and systems that administer the vaccine and in individual beliefs about vaccine safety. In our COVID experience, all three are in play when looking at individual decisions to accept a COVID vaccine, delay it, or refuse it altogether.

For many years local, state, and federal public health agencies have tried to make it as easy as possible for parents to vaccinate their children and for adults to receive their recommended immunizations. The provision of vaccines at no cost to patients, the inclusion of pharmacy partners able to administer vaccines, and state laws that expand the number of health professionals licensed to administer vaccines have all been successful strategies to make vaccines more convenient. A focus on convenience has been a significant part of federal and state COVID vaccine rollout plans by employing pharmacies as well as creating alternative vaccination sites such as sports arenas or mall parking lots. Health officials and their partners have made it possible for most Americans to be vaccinated in their communities.

Making COVID vaccine convenient was a complicated endeavor. As describe earlier, jurisdictions made a Herculean effort to make vaccines both free and available to all Americans. While important, convenience is just one aspect of vaccine hesitancy. Making vaccines available (easy to access, no cost to patients) does not mean individuals will choose to get vaccinated. The United States spent billions to develop COVID vaccines and get them to practically every street corner in America, but still a sizable percentage of the population has yet to be vaccinated. Addressing complacency and confidence proved to be much more difficult in the COVID vaccine campaign, largely because complacency and confidence involve individual feelings and beliefs that shape an individual's health behaviors.

One of the most frequent criticisms of the US national response to COVID was the inconsistent messaging concerning the severity of the illness and the health risks associated with infection. In January and February of 2020, the first few months of the pandemic in the United States, many politicians downplayed the risks associated with COVID, comparing it to a mild case of seasonal flu or a bad cold. But very little was known about the virus at the time. As President Trump reassured the public that COVID was not going to be all that bad, China constructed a 1,000-bed hospital in 10 days. Toward the end of January 2021, China locked down millions of citizens in the city of Wuhan and several other locations to stop the virus from spreading.[62] Obviously, the emerging virus was potentially more severe than a mild cold or flu.

As the virus spread and more was learned about it, it became clear that COVID illness could affect multiple organ systems and could also cause lasting symptoms, or "long COVID," that we are only now beginning to understand more completely.[63] As health officials learned more about the virus and its impact, it became increasingly clear that COVID was spreading asymptomatically around the globe and severity was indeed high, especially among older persons and those with existing medical conditions. But the reality of COVID for many Americans was still far away, especially those not living in the East or West Coast population centers most affected early in COVID's spread.

In earlier chapters of this book, we illustrated how President Trump and other federal officials publicly downplayed the risks associated with the novel virus, stating in daily briefings and press conferences that everything was under control and that COVID was no big deal. These public reassurances contradicted, however, what the president and others knew early in the pandemic: COVID was indeed serious, with catastrophic potential to infect millions and kill hundreds of thousands. In his interviews with Bob Woodward in March 2021, Trump acknowledged that COVID was deadly, but he stated, "I wanted to always play it down . . . I still like playing it down, because I don't want to create a panic."[64,65]

Those early months set in motion two dueling descriptions of the reality of COVID's severity. One narrative, shared by health care professionals and public health officials as they learned more about the virus and its impact, suggested coronavirus was a serious threat to the health of all Americans and the risk was so great that conditions merited business and school closures, as well as other disruptions to everyday life. The other narrative, stated publicly by President Trump and his supporters, was that COVID was little more than the common cold or flu and was a virus that would miraculously disappear—indeed, President Trump stated on February 27, 2020, that "one day it's like a miracle, it will disappear."[66]

Those supportive of the Trump narrative downplayed the need to take extra precautions or require business closures, questioned how cases were being counted or defined to minimize the numbers of them, and even began to say that COVID was a hoax, a fiction being portrayed to undermine the president's leadership and reelection bid. Even after his own bout of COVID, for which the president required hospitalization at Washington's Walter Reed Medical Center, he continued to minimize the risk of COVID's severity, telling American's he felt better post-COVID than he had felt "in 20 years," and exhorting the public not to let COVID "dominate your lives."[67]

The unfortunate consequence of these two narratives was the politicization of COVID response: studies in the summer of 2020 showed that Republicans were less likely to perceive COVID as a threat to their health than were Democrats, who viewed it a significant threat. In their 2022 article "Prevention Is Political," researchers Kiviniemi, Orom, Hay, and Waters found that Republican or Democratic political party affiliation predicted

COVID risk protection behavior, including vaccination, stating, "The more strongly one identified as a Republican, the less risk one perceived to oneself from SARS-CoV-2/COVID-19 and the less risk one perceived other people faced. Moreover, those identifying as more strongly Republican engaged in fewer preventive behaviors."[68] Their research confirmed earlier studies that found a relationship between higher COVID morbidity and mortality in US counties that voted for Trump and higher vaccine hesitancy and refusal among Republicans than Democrats.[69,70]

That one's chance of being vaccinated could be predicted by who you voted for marked a sad day in America's public health history. Public health, while often political, was rarely so partisan. Diseases do not care who one votes for, nor do viruses select their hosts by political affiliation. And while in earlier studies researchers had observed differences between vaccination status by political party, the magnitude of the association in COVID was indeed unparalleled.

In March 2021, the public health think tank de Beaumont Foundation engaged GOP pollster and communications consultant Dr. Frank Luntz to help inform steps public health professionals could take to address the partisan divide in vaccine hesitancy.[71,72,73] In a nationwide survey of 1,000 Republicans who voted for President Trump, vaccine complacency was the top reason for Republicans not getting vaccinated. The survey found that the most hesitant Republicans did not see COVID as a serious threat to their health, and in some cases they viewed the vaccine as potentially more dangerous than COVID itself. The survey also showed that respondents were not opposed to vaccines overall—most reported they had received childhood and young adult vaccines, and on average around 63% of the group accepted flu shots—but rather, they questioned the reason to get vaccinated in the first place, given their low perceived risk of serious illness (survey data from "The Language of GOP Vaccine Confidence," an internal PowerPoint presentation, shared with the authors by Frank Luntz, DPhil and de Beaumont, March 30, 2021).

The research by Dr. Luntz and the de Beaumont Foundation also showed that the most effective way to address vaccine complacency among this group was not to try to convince these Republican voters of the severity of COVID or the consequences of not being vaccinated but instead to stress the benefits of being vaccinated and how it will expand their individual freedom and thus "allow me to live life as freely as it was before" (from "The Language of GOP Vaccine Confidence," an internal PowerPoint presentation, shared with the authors by Frank Luntz, DPhil, and de Beaumont, March 30, 2021). They also found that the most trusted messengers for the vaccine message were physicians known and trusted by the individuals themselves. This was counter to prevalent messaging to address complacency that attempted to either shame the unvaccinated or stressed the likelihood of unvaccinated individuals getting ill, or even worse, dying. These messages also came from politicians and government officials, thereby adding to mistrust.

For example, on December 20, 2021, Chief of Staff Ron Klain retweeted a White House tweet with the comment that "the truth is the truth"[74]:

> We are intent on not letting Omicron disrupt work and school for the vaccinated. You've done the right thing, and we will get through this.
> For the unvaccinated, you're looking at a winter of severe illness and death for yourselves, your families, and the hospitals you may soon overwhelm.[74]

Unfortunately, according to the research by Luntz and de Beaumont, this was exactly the wrong message and wrong messenger to communicate to a large percentage of vaccine-complacent Republicans. While their research offered immensely useful insights, to what extent it was applied in the communities that needed it most remains unclear.

Over the last two years, individual perceptions about the severity of COVID changed greatly as more was learned about the virus, more people experienced infections, and vaccines helped lessen disease severity. According to longitudinal surveys conducted by Morning Consult, in March 2020 some 39% of Americans believed that the coronavirus "is a severe health risk in their local community," and by July 2022 just 14% believed the same.[75] Changing policies, such as lifting restrictions on mask wearing in public transportation or the CDC's move to report on county-based "community levels" of COVID transmission and hospital capacity versus individual cases, changed how individuals perceived their own risk of COVID and weighed that with the benefits of vaccination.[76] While new variants and rising cases have concerned public health officials, vaccination rates have not increased significantly as a result. For the time being, vaccine complacency remains a challenge for health officials eager to promote continued vaccination but facing a public, or at least a sizable percentage of the public, that believe COVID is not that big a deal.

Addressing how individual's perceive risk of disease and understanding how perceived risk shapes health behaviors is complicated. What we have seen with COVID vaccine complacency tracks with overall vaccine complacency more broadly: a significant percentage of the population is willing to forgo a potentially lifesaving vaccine because of subjective perceptions of risk that are not necessarily factual or science based but are, rather, influenced by political views, social networks, and personal values and beliefs.

To address complacency, however, messages that stress disease severity or suggest that individual perceptions of risk are wrong may not be all that successful with certain audiences. Instead, understanding what is driving the complacency is the key to moving people from hesitancy to acceptance. This is an insight many public health officials learned throughout the pandemic—for example, Dr. Anne Zink, Alaska's chief medical officer, wrote in an opinion piece in the *Washington Post* in October 2021, "Eventually, as occurred in many other rural states, our vaccination effort stalled. Hesitancy and misinformation made many people underestimate the risk of covid-19 infections and overestimate the risk from the coronavirus vaccines."[77] Many Alaskans, and many other Americans, got sick and died as a result.

In a June 10, 2022, oral interview with us, Dr. Tom Frieden also picked up on the unique challenges promoting vaccines in rural America. He told us, "One of the things I've tried to emphasize is public health understands that when there are questions about vaccination from Black or Hispanic communities, people deserve to have their concerns listened to and addressed. And I think public health has been less attuned to that for rural white communities." Indeed, pockets of the most vaccine-hesitant Americans are now rural, white communities, not because vaccines are less available in those places, but because vaccine confidence and trust in public health messengers is lower.

VACCINE CONFIDENCE AND BUILDING TRUST

In October 2019, CDC announced a new vaccination promotion campaign: Vaccinate with Confidence.[78] The campaign, complete with a logo comprising blue and green Band-Aids joined together at the bottom to create a V shape, was the most recent of several efforts to work with state and local health immunization programs to build support for vaccines, especially in communities where vaccine hesitancy and refusal had begun to take hold. The campaign's aim was to combine CDC's "existing work with new investments, partnerships, and activities to protect communities at risk and strengthen public trust in the life-saving protection of vaccines."[79] Crucial to the campaign was the element of building trust between vaccine providers, their patients, and their communities as a strategy to promote vaccine confidence. In addition to sharing fact-based information about vaccine safety and efficacy, the campaign was designed to promote meaningful, transparent engagement between community members and public health authorities.

The campaign's focus on trust building and transparency signaled a welcome recognition of the need to build trusting partnerships between governmental public health officials, clinicians, and community members. In many previous efforts to address vaccine hesitancy, lack of knowledge about vaccines was seen as the main reason for an individual's vaccine hesitancy.[79] Efforts to move individuals from hesitancy to confidence focused on sharing facts and data about vaccine effectiveness, most often by health care professionals, who are viewed as the most trusted sources of health information in many communities. But information deficit is not always the primary reason someone delays or refuses vaccination, and telling individuals vaccines are safe and sharing more science with them does not move them toward vaccine acceptance. In addition to providing fact-based materials about why vaccines are safe and effective, more recent public health efforts have begun to address a far more difficult cause of vaccine hesitancy: lack of trust.

Trust is essential to vaccine acceptance. If you do not trust the science that guides how a vaccine is made, the process by which it is manufactured, the industry that makes it, the public health or health care professionals who administer it, or the organizations those professionals work for, you are far more likely to delay or avoid vaccination. No amount of information about the basics of immunology or the safety of modern vaccine production is going to build trust among individuals who mistrust the health care system delivering the vaccine or distrust the motives of government and industries for developing them. Lack of trust has been a monumental hurdle for health officials to overcome in their efforts to vaccinate Americans against COVID and continues to challenge public health professionals nationwide today.

When it comes to who Americans trust to provide reliable information on COVID vaccines, the good news is that people's own doctors top the list, with 85% of adults telling researchers they trust their personal doctor "a great deal" or "a fair amount."[80] Similarly, 83% of parents say they trust their child's pediatrician to provide them with reliable information about the COVID-19 vaccines. The same research also reported that majorities of workers trust their employer (77%), insured adults trust their health insurance company (73%), and majorities trust their local public health department (68%) for this information. But signaling concern, only two-thirds trust COVID-19 vaccine information from the CDC (64%) or the Food and Drug Administration (FDA; 62%), and about half of adults trust their state government officials (54%), Dr. Anthony Fauci (53%), and President Joe Biden (49%).[80]

Public health efforts to increase COVID vaccine confidence have been stymied by two very different perspectives rooted in distrust. The first perspective, that COVID vaccine production was rushed and that the process created unsafe vaccines, has led many to distrust governmental public health agency efforts to promote vaccines and has led to many myths, mistruths, and conspiracies about COVID vaccine development and vaccine safety. The second perspective, that the organizations and institutions that developed and promoted COVID vaccines cannot be trusted by people of color, and especially by Black Americans, is rooted in the collective historical trauma created by medical experimentation and exploitation experienced by many Black, brown, and Native American people. It is also justified and confirmed by the lived experience of discrimination and racism in current interactions with the health care and public health systems.

The typical vaccine development process takes years to complete and requires enormous amounts of data to meet strict regulatory requirements for safety and efficacy. COVID vaccine development, however, was completed in record time through a series of creative bureaucratic changes and efficiencies because the COVID emergency allowed manufacturers to enroll patient's conduct clinical trials, and begin manufacturing simultaneously.

Questions about the safety of expedited vaccine review and approval, and the politicization of the emergency use authorization process, became so acute by August and early September 2020 that some state and territorial health officials publicly shared concerns that the review process might be purposefully accelerated to boost the president's reelection at the expense of assuring vaccine safety. Former president of the Association of

State and Territorial Health Officials (ASTHO) and Pennsylvania's secretary of health Dr. Rachel Levine, now assistant secretary for health in the Biden administration, described consulting with vaccine experts in her state, including Dr. Paul Offit, to assess the safety issues associated with expedited review of clinical trial data. Health officials reported that several governors were considering establishing their own COVID vaccine safety review panels because they did not trust the FDA's process.

In addition, the National Medical Association, the medical society of Black physicians in the United States, similarly stated it would review the FDA's clinical trial data before recommending the Pfizer and Moderna vaccines to patients. Subsequently, after an expert review, the National Medical Association supported the FDA's emergency use authorization and recommended vaccinations in an advisory issued on December 21, 2020.[81]

On September 3, 2020, ASTHO issued a press statement in which Dr. Levine called on FDA commissioner Dr. Stephen Hahn and Dr. Anthony Fauci of the National Institutes of Health (NIH) to clarify statements made indicating the FDA may authorize a COVID vaccine before the completion of Phase 3 clinical trials. Dr. Levine stated:

> Our nation's health officials are concerned by recent statements from FDA Commissioner Hahn and NIAID Director Fauci indicating they would consider authorizing the use of a COVID-19 vaccine prior to the completion of phase 3 clinical trials. The safety and efficacy of vaccines is paramount to protecting the health of the American public and to building confidence in our state and territorial immunization programs . . .
>
> In these unprecedented times, the federal government must uphold a key principle of medical practice to "do no harm." We look forward to partnering with FDA, NIH, CDC, and other federal agencies to provide insight and guidance, utilize state and local experience with previous mass vaccination campaigns, and support a timeline that is grounded in ethical decision-making.[82]

To address these concerns, the ASTHO Executive Committee requested principals from HHS, FDA, NIH, and CDC to join a teleconference to assure public health leaders that the emergency use authorization review process was free of political interference and that the FDA was following all required protocols to confirm vaccine safety. A teleconference was held on September 10, 2020, and attended by ASTHO's leadership and HHS principals Dr. Brett Giroir, assistant secretary of health; Surgeon General Jerome Adams; Commissioner Stephen Hahn; Dr. Anthony Fauci, NIH's National Institute of Allergy and Infectious Diseases director; CDC director Dr. Robert Redfield; and Ms. Cecily Waters from the Office of the Assistant Secretary for Preparedness and Response.

At the opening of the meeting Dr. Levine stated, "Science is science. And you can't rush science" (author's own notes, "ASTHO/HHS Leadership Meeting. September 10, 2020. Meeting Notes") summarizing the concerns of state health officials about the accelerated timeline. Federal officials on the call explained the FDA's review process and were emphatic that there were no plans to rush vaccine despite directives to states to prepare for vaccination rollout as early as November 1, 2020. Stating that regular leader-level communication would be essential to addressing shared concerns in the weeks ahead, Dr. Levine proposed a weekly meeting of HHS principals and state health officers to coordinate efforts and address concerns. Dr. Giroir stated his commitment as assistant secretary of health to such regular meetings, especially to "repair the situation and have good communication," sharing that communication is important for credibility, alignment, and the public's health (author's own notes, "ASTHO/HHS Leadership Meeting. September 10, 2020. Meeting Notes"). Despite attempts to schedule such meetings, however, none were held in follow-up.

Eager to develop COVID vaccines and get the nation's economy back on track, President Trump relentlessly criticized the FDA for its lengthy authorization and safety review process despite his earlier skepticism about vaccines. Accusing the agency's "deep state" civil servants of trying to sabotage his reelection bid by withholding their authorization until after Election Day,[83] Trump pushed the FDA to rush its vaccine review process, raising questions about whether an authorized vaccine would be safe.

In public reporting on the president's remarks, Dr. Peter Marks, head of the FDA's Center for Biologics Evaluation and Research (CBER), stated he would resign if he believed any safety corners were being cut, saying this as a signal to health officials and the public that new COVID vaccines were not being used to score political points at the expense of the public's health.[84] Dr. Marks subsequently became a regular participant on ASTHO's state and territorial health officials' teleconferences updating health officers on the approval process and answering questions about clinical trials and safety and efficacy studies being monitored by CBER and the FDA. To this day, he remains head of CBER at the FDA.

Unfortunately, however, the perception that vaccine development was being rushed and safety measures were not being followed was enough to raise skepticism about COVID vaccine safety well before the vaccines were administered. In December 2020, the month vaccines were first rolled out in the United States, the Kaiser Family Foundation's Vaccine Monitor survey found that 34% of Americans surveyed said they would take a COVID vaccine as soon as they could get it, but 39% stated they would take a "wait and see" approach before they got it.[85] And while the wait-and-see group began to shrink in the first few months, down to 17% in March 2020, many still did not trust the review process and wanted to observe how vaccination played out before opting to get their COVID shot. It was clear that developing broad confidence in vaccines developed in record time and at warp speed was going to be incredibly challenging.

The myth that COVID vaccines are unsafe because of the speed of their development is just one of the many controversies surrounding COVID vaccines. Health officials have dealt with false reports that COVID vaccines make individuals magnetic to create human 5G (and even 6G) cell phone towers, that COVID vaccines contain microchips to identify and track you, that it is the vaccine that is producing variants, that COVID vaccine can make you infertile, that mRNA vaccines change your DNA, or that COVID vaccines cause autism or other developmental delays. These conspiracy theories and myths, generally spread via social media influencers eager to increase their click rates and corresponding advertising revenue on multiple online platforms such as Twitter, Instagram, or Facebook, raised enough concern and doubt about vaccine safety that many Americans chose to delay or refuse COVID vaccination altogether.[86,87,88,89]

In November 2021, the de Beaumont Foundation released new research showing that people who said social media was an influential source of information about COVID were 16% less likely to report that they had received at least one dose of a COVID vaccine.[90] Overall, respondents to the foundation's poll said that television news or their own doctor was their most influential source of information about COVID, "but those who said that social media is a major source were far more likely to believe false and misleading statements about COVID-19."[91] Dr. Frank Luntz, who had conducted the poll for de Beaumont, said, "These results show more clearly than ever that the people who rely on social media as a primary source of information about COVID-19—and those who use social media most frequently—are most likely to believe false information. Worse yet, it proves that people who most frequently share social media information are most likely to be misinformed."[91]

Such social media-fueled vaccine hesitancy led to increasing numbers of cases, and COVID deaths, in many states, including Mississippi, where state officials had to request federal support to run a field hospital out of a medical center parking deck because the hospital was so overrun. Frustrated by the lack of vaccine uptake and online conspiracies driving hesitancy in his state, former Mississippi state health officer Dr. Thomas Dobbs stated at a press conference in April 2021:

> We should not be here, y'all. This is not necessary. Too many people are getting information from wrong sources . . . These Facebook conspiratorial lists are going to spread and run, and have no accountability for the people who are dying, and we're here, picking up the mess.[1]

Dr. Dobbs's sentiment characterized the feelings of many health officers who witnessed similar surges in illness and death in their own states because of online disinformation, misinformation, and lack of trust.

Research by the Center for Countering Digital Hate, a nonprofit think tank that monitors online hate speech and vaccine dis- and misinformation, found that the majority of anti-COVID vaccine internet influencers have employed a shared strategy to increase vaccine hesitancy and decrease trust in vaccines. This strategy, described in the center's report "The Anti-vaxx Playbook," has three parts.[92] First, anti-vaxx social media influencers spread the myth that COVID's severity has been overstated by public health officials and COVID is not dangerous. Second, they undermine trust in vaccine safety by spreading the myth that COVID vaccines (and other vaccines) are dangerous. Third, they generate mistrust of physicians, scientists, and public health officials by claiming that they receive financial or professional gain from COVID, a myth spread by President Trump himself. At a campaign rally on October 30, 2020, the president stated, "Our doctors get more money if somebody dies from COVID . . . So what they do is they say, 'I'm sorry, but, you know, everybody dies of COVID.'"[93]

With a plethora of information and misinformation about COVID vaccines available online, individuals searching for information can find a post or a link to practically any source that supports their worldview and can easily share it with others. The vast amount of vaccine misinformation and disinformation available online creates a massive threat for public health officials to counter: most health departments or public health authorities do not have the time, resources, or technology resources to mount as robust of an online presence as the anti-vaxxers.[94,95,96,97]

Regarding misinformation, Claire Hannan, MPH, told us in our March 17, 2022, oral interview that "as soon as you disprove one thing, there's a new thing that comes out. So, there's always gonna be that angle to misinformation, but I think you have to continue to put the right information out and you have to continue to encourage family members. I think family members are really the trusted source right now. You have to continue to address the misinformation, but it's never going to fully go away." To build trust in vaccines and help create vaccine confidence, many have called on social media platforms to better monitor and regulate the COVID vaccine information being posted on their sites. While effective in some cases, the sheer volume of such information makes it difficult to comprehensively police. For overstretched public health agencies, mounting an effective counterresponse to such posts is practically impossible.

Furthermore, the speed at which misinformation can travel via the internet is unprecedented, although the concepts about the speed of misinformation are present throughout history. Mark Twain is sometimes credited as saying, "A lie can get halfway around the world before the truth can put on its shoes."[98] This maxim echoes an earlier statement by Jonathan Swift that "falsehood flies, and the truth comes limping after it; so that when men come to be undeceiv'd, it is too late; the jest is over, and the tale has had its effect."[99] Both statements echo an even more ancient observation from Greek historian Thucydides, who wrote in his *History of the Peloponnesian War* in 431 BC that "most people, in fact, will not take the trouble in finding out the truth, but are much more inclined to accept the first story they hear."[100] So the challenges are not new, but in the internet age a lie can get all the way around the world three times before efforts to share the truth can even be organized.

Such a counteroffensive, however, is sorely needed. In a 2021 commentary "COVID Vaccines: Time to Confront Anti-vax Aggression," Dr. Peter Hotez makes the case that public health officials need a new strategy to build trust in vaccines, a position we endorse wholeheartedly:

I have a long-standing disagreement with many of my US public-health colleagues. I admire their commitment to disease prevention, but when I ask for a more direct way to counter anti-vaccine aggression, I'm told, "that's not our approach; confrontation gives them a plat-form and oxygen." In my opinion, this attitude reflects a time when we had dial-up modems. Today, the anti-vaccine empire has hundreds of websites and perhaps 58 million followers on social media. The bad guys are winning, in part because health agencies either underes-timate or deny the reach of anti-science forces, and are ill-equipped to counter it.[96]

With all the resources being invested in COVID vaccine, the creation of a national center to counter online vaccine misinformation could have easily been a funded priority alongside vaccine development and administration. Now public health officials are left playing catch-up—or worse, in Hotez's words, letting the "bad guys" win.[96]

While conspiracy theories, disinformation, and myths about rushed vaccine develop-ment contributed to vaccine hesitancy and refusal, other significant concerns that eroded vaccine confidence and trust in vaccines were apprehensions raised by people of color, especially Black Americans, about vaccine safety as related to past medical experimenta-tion. Medical experimentation on people of color is a shameful part of America's history that includes multiple examples of dubious research ethics, if not outright unethical research methods.[101] The most widely known example of unethical treatment of Black Americans in medical research, though certainly not the only case, was the infamous "Tuskegee Study of Untreated Syphilis in the Negro Male."[102,103] Conducted in Macon County, Alabama, by the US Public Health Service and the CDC, researchers followed a cohort of Black men with syphilis who thought they were receiving treatment for "bad blood,"[103] when in fact they were receiving no treatment at all, even after it was estab-lished that penicillin could be used effectively to treat them. Over the course of the research period, participants were in many cases prevented from receiving treatment.

When a whistleblower drew attention to the study and its harmful and unethical treat-ment of research participants in 1972, a tremendous public outcry ended the project. To this day, however, the legacy of distrust in government and in health care and public health research the Tuskegee study engendered in the Black community lives on. In her commentary on the experience of being a patient in a COVID vaccine clinical trial pub-lished in *The Lancet*, Dr. Kimberly Manning, Emory School of Medicine's associate vice chair for diversity equity, reflected on the Tuskegee study but also on the broader impact of racism and discrimination:

There are trust issues when it comes to African Americans and the US health-care system. There is also a justified fear that our human lives might be dispensable in exchange for sci-entific discovery benefiting those with privilege and who are white. The historical basis for this, which began long before the untreated syphilis study in Macon County, underscores a larger, ongoing issue—the value of Black lives. In the Antebellum period, it was the millions tortured through chattel slavery as property. Post Reconstruction, there was state-sanctioned convict leasing followed by Jim Crow laws and domestic terrorism. The uncovering of the disturbing events in the Tuskegee study was no more than another chapter over centuries in

US history. It is a story that continues with the deaths of unarmed Black Americans, mass incarceration, the achievement gap, and the astounding health disparities seen every day and now amplified by COVID-19. All of it is intertwined.[104(p1482)]

Rahmell Peebles, a Black New York City resident, put it simply in an interview with the Associated Press in April 2020: "I've just been conditioned not to trust . . . If we got to a place where the government says, 'OK, now it's time to take a vaccine,' then I'm definitely going to be skeptical of their intentions."[2]

COVID has disproportionately affected Black Americans and other racial and ethnic minorities, acting as a magnifying glass on glaring disparities the nation faces between white and nonwhite Americans. Pre-COVID disparities in vaccine rates demonstrate the ongoing challenge: although the federal government's Vaccines for Children program dramatically reduced many racial and ethnic vaccine coverage disparities, Black Americans still have lower rates than whites on many childhood and adult vaccination rates. While some of the vaccine rate disparity may be due to convenience factors such as access to health care, lack of health insurance, or cost (among those not eligible for the Vaccines for Children program), some is certainly attributable to individuals avoiding care as a result of having experienced racial discrimination and thus lacking trust in the health care and public health systems. Effective strategies to address vaccine hesitancy among Black Americans, as well as Hispanic and Native and Indigenous Americans, need to focus not only on addressing barriers to vaccine access but also increasing trust in the systems that administer vaccines overall.[105]

Washington Post columnist Michele Norris proposed on December 9, 2020, just days before Sandra Lindsay, a Black nurse in New York, received the first COVID vaccination outside a clinical trial in the United States, that an "Operation Build Trust" be developed to address vaccine confidence among Black and brown Americans with the same urgency Operation Warp Speed used to accelerate the development of the vaccines.[106] Anticipating low vaccination rates among Black Americans because of distrust and the lived experiences of racism, not conspiracy, she wrote:

> "Vaccine hesitancy" from Black Americans is different from an "anti-vaxxer" stance. It's not that Black Americans don't believe in vaccines. They don't trust a public health system that has in too many cases engaged in grievous harm by experimenting on Black bodies without consent or ignoring the specific needs of Black people.[107]

Structural racism, a term used to refer to the "totality of ways that societies foster racial discrimination through mutually reinforcing systems of housing, education, employment, earning, benefits, credit, media, health care and criminal justice,"[107] creates distrust. If you believe that a system does not have your best interest in mind—or worse, you believe you are inferior to other groups in the society because of your race—or it wants to harm you, you are far less likely to want to interact with that system or trust that system in the first place.

In a study that looked at the relationship between race, vaccination rates, and the level of structural racism in states, Siegel and colleagues found Black and Hispanic Americans had lower COVID vaccination rates in almost all the states in their analysis.[105] The researchers also found that the magnitude of the difference between white and nonwhite vaccination rates could be explained in part by the level of structural racism in the state: those states with a higher state racism index had fewer vaccinations among Blacks and Hispanics. In other words, COVID vaccine hesitancy among Blacks and Hispanic Americans was higher in states with higher structural racism scores, most likely the result of long-established inequities in how different groups had been treated over the course of the state's history and their experience with the public health and health care systems.

Developing trust requires a great deal of time, attention, and investment and is most definitely difficult to accomplish in the middle of all the exigencies of a pandemic, but trust is essential to ending one. To help build trust and increase vaccine confidence among Black Americans, a significant strategy implemented by public health agencies was to partner with institutions and organizations that had a track record of established trust within communities. Public health agencies reached out to faith leaders and clergy of Black churches to help increase vaccination rates as established and trusted voices in the Black community. Black physicians and public health leaders wrote newspaper editorials and opinions and recorded videos to help build vaccine confidence. Established community groups and nonprofits that work with Black, brown, and Native American residents were funded to do outreach, share information, and promote trust in the organizations administering COVID vaccines.

These strategies worked. Researchers examining vaccine hesitancy in the first six months of the COVID vaccine rollout found that Black vaccine hesitancy decreased faster than white vaccine hesitancy, largely the result of increased belief that getting vaccinated was important to protecting themselves and their families.[108] While a gap remains in many states between the percentage of the white population vaccinated and the percentage of the Black and Hispanic population vaccinated, the successful engagement of community leaders and trusted community groups in increasing COVID vaccine confidence is a bright spot in the COVID response.

THE IMPORTANCE OF TRUST

Recent research by the COVID-19 National Preparedness Collaborators looking at how well, or how poorly, different countries around the world were able to control COVID infections found that societies that had better vaccine coverage and fewer deaths exhibited high levels of social cohesion and high levels of trust in government and interpersonal trust.[109] In many ways, this finding is so simple as to be obvious: countries in which citizens trusted each other to do the right thing and look out for each other, and trusted government information and actions to stop the virus, did better in the pandemic.

But the finding is remarkable, given assumptions we make about a country's resources, the adequacy of the country's health care system, and the sociodemographics of its population. We would generally expect the richest countries to do the best because of their ability to spend resources on the problem, or we suppose that countries with the best health care systems would do better in a pandemic than countries without a public health system. But the simple fact that while resources matter, trust—the simple, interpersonal act of believing someone else has your best interests in mind—matters more. The researchers found that countries with high trust in government and interpersonal trust had lower COVID infection rates. In addition, high trust in government and interpersonal trust in high- and middle-income countries was associated with higher COVID vaccination coverage. In modeling the importance of trust to preventing COVID infection, the researchers state:

> If these modelled associations were to be causal, an increase in trust of governments such that all countries had societies that attained at least the amount of trust in government or interpersonal trust measured in Denmark, which is in the 75th percentile across these spectrums, might have reduced global infections by 12.9% (5.7–17.8) for government trust and 40.3% (24.3–51.4) for interpersonal trust.[109(p1489)]

They conclude their study with the also simple but exceedingly complex recommendation that "governments should invest in risk communication and community engagement strategies to boost the confidence that individuals have in government guidance in public health crises, especially in settings with historically low levels of government and interpersonal trust."[109(p1509)] Michele Norris was on to something when she suggested Operation Build Trust as a companion effort to Operation Warp Speed.

Research spearheaded by the Harvard Opinion Research Program in partnership with ASTHO and the National Public Health Information Coalition has carefully examined public trust in governmental public health agencies throughout the COVID response ("Enhancing Trust in Public Health: When Recommendations Change," an internal PowerPoint presentation of survey data collection, March 13–April 12, 2022, shared with authors).[110] Key findings from a research brief summarizing public opinion survey data from April 2022 demonstrate that those who were most trusting of public health agencies were individuals who viewed those agencies as making science-based decisions, while those least trusting of public health agencies believed health officials made recommendations due to private-sector or political influence.

In related research conducted by Harvard's T.H. Chan School of Public Health and the Robert Wood Johnson Foundation in May 2021, researchers found that with regard to health-related recommendations, the public was far more trusting of health care providers, including nurses and physicians, than they were of governmental institutions such as public health agencies.[111] Only 52% of survey respondents trusted the CDC a "Great deal/Quite a lot," 44% trusted their local health department a "Great deal/Quite a lot," and 41% trusted their state health department a "Great deal/Quite a lot."[111(p5)] The researchers also found the public was divided on the job performance of their jurisdiction's governmental public health agencies, noting:

> When it comes to rating the job performance of their own state and local health departments, the public is also divided. About half of adults (49%) say their state health department is doing an excellent or good job at protecting the public from health threats and preventing illness, including responding to the Covid-19 outbreak, while 51% say it is doing a fair or poor job. Similarly, a slight majority of adults (53%) say their local health department is doing an excellent or good job at protecting the public from health threats and preventing illness, including responding to the Covid-19 outbreak, while 46% say it is doing a fair or poor job.[111(p8)]

What has stalled our nation's vaccination rate and has certainly led to needless suffering and preventable deaths due to COVID has been a lack of social cohesion and a lack of trust by a large segment of the American population. COVID could have been an event that unified a divided nation. Instead, it further split us apart despite the admirable attempts of so many leaders. Divisiveness, not togetherness, characterized the months and years we have lived with COVID. Conspiracy theories and disinformation cast doubt on the amazing scientific advances that were made to get COVID vaccines to market at record speed and disparaged the professionals administering the vaccines. Suspicion, doubt, and mistrust generated enough vaccine hesitancy and refusal in the country that to this day America has not been able to adequately control the COVID pandemic.

Building trust, therefore, must be a key aspect of COVID recovery efforts and future pandemic preparedness plans. Developing sincere, empathetic, trauma-informed, and authentic connections between public health agencies and the communities they serve should be a priority for all public health professionals.[112]

Commenting on the study comparing countries' levels of trust with their COVID response outcomes,[109] *New York Times* opinion columnist Ezra Klein summed it up this way: "You know what's better than a vaccine mandate? A society that doesn't need one."[113] While this aspiration would be extremely difficult to accomplish in a divisive environment that fosters suspicion and conspiracy over trust and confidence, one would hope that leaders facing future pandemics could, at least temporarily, put aside partisan differences and promote social cohesion and unity. Indeed, the more we trust each other, the better our chances of ending a pandemic the next time.

REFERENCES

1. Mitropoulos A. Field hospital opens in parking garage as Mississippi sees "skyrocketing" crush of COVID patients. *ABC News*. August 13, 2021. Available at: https://abcnews.go.com/Health/field-hospital-opens-parking-garage-mississippi-sees-skyrocketing/story?id=79433418. Accessed September 17, 2022.

2. Morrison A, Reeves J. Amid coronavirus pandemic, Black mistrust of medicine looms. *AP News*. April 5, 2020. Available at: https://apnews.com/article/health-us-news-ap-top-news-ms-state-wire-virus-outbreak-5aa41953a211049f53a62df18b6f7b87. Accessed September 17, 2022.

3. National Center for Health Statistics. Daily updates of totals by week and state from the National Vital Statistics System. Centers for Disease Control and Prevention. August 12, 2022. Available at: https://www.cdc.gov/nchs/nvss/index.htm. Accessed September 17, 2022.

4. Schumaker E. Long lines for COVID-19 vaccines build in Florida, Tennessee, Puerto Rico. *ABC News*. December 31, 2020. Available at: https://abcnews.go.com/US/long-lines-covid-19-vaccines-build-florida-tennessee/story?id=74988405. Accessed September 17, 2022.

5. Holcombe M. Florida seniors face long lines and a haphazard registration system to get COVID-19 vaccines. *CNN*. January 7, 2021. Available at: https://www.cnn.com/2021/01/07/us/florida-coronavirus-vaccine-rollout/index.html. Accessed September 23, 2022.

6. Goldhill O, St. Fleur N. "There absolutely will be a black market": how the rich and privileged can skip the line for COVID-19 vaccines. *STAT*. December 3, 2020. Available at: https://www.statnews.com/2020/12/03/how-rich-and-privileged-can-skip-the-line-for-covid19-vaccines. Accessed September 23, 2022.

7. Nelson LJ, Lau M. The wealthy scramble for COVID-19 vaccines: "If I donate $25,000 . . . would that help me?" *Los Angeles Times*. December 18, 2020. Available at: https://www.latimes.com/california/story/2020-12-18/wealthy-patients-scramble-covid-19-vaccine. Accessed September 23, 2022.

8. Hamel L, Kearney A, Kirzinger A, Lopes L, Munana C, Brodie M. KFF health tracking poll—September 2020: top issues in 2020 election, the role of misinformation, and views on a potential coronavirus vaccine. KFF. September 10, 2020. Available at: https://www.kff.org/coronavirus-covid-19/report/kff-health-tracking-poll-september-2020. Accessed September 17, 2022.

9. The White House. Fact sheet: President Biden to announce all Americans to be eligible for vaccinations by May 1, puts the nation on a path to get closer to normal by July 4th. March 11, 2021. Available at: https://www.whitehouse.gov/briefing-room/statements-releases/2021/03/11/fact-sheet-president-biden-to-announce-all-americans-to-be-eligible-for-vaccinations-by-may-1-puts-the-nation-on-a-path-to-get-closer-to-normal-by-july-4th. Accessed September 23, 2022.

10. Ritchie H, Mathieu E, Rodés-Guirao L, et al. Coronavirus pandemic (COVID-19). Our World in Data. 2020. Updated daily. Available at: https://ourworldindata.org/coronavirus. Accessed September 17, 2022.

11. World Health Organization. Ten threats to global health in 2019. Available at: https://www.who.int/news-room/spotlight/ten-threats-to-global-health-in-2019. Accessed September 23, 2022.

12. Ochieng N, Chidambaram P, Musumeci MB. Nursing facility staffing shortages during the COVID-19 pandemic. KFF. February 17, 2022. Updated April 4, 2022. Available at:

https://www.kff.org/coronavirus-covid-19/issue-brief/nursing-facility-staffing-shortages-during-the-covid-19-pandemic. Accessed September 23, 2022.

13. Dumyati G, Jump RLP, Gaur S. Mandating COVID-19 vaccine for nursing home staff: an ethical obligation. *J Am Med Dir Assoc.* 2021;22(10):1967–1968. doi:10.1016/j.jamda.2021.08.017.

14. sikaMusi S (@SizweLo). Bill Gates is launching implantable chips which will be used to show whether a person has been tested and vaccinated for Corona. These microchips will dissolve under the skin, leaving identification 'quantum dots'. These implants and can also be used as a form of ID. Twitter. Pic.twitter.com/5vibjltyn1. Posted March 25, 2020. Available at: https://twitter.com/SizweLo/status/1242753291605495810?ref_src=twsrc%5Etfw%7Ctwcamp%5Etweetembed%7Ctwterm%5E1242753291605495810%7Ctwgr%5E%7Ctwcon%5Es1_&ref_url=https%3A%2F%2Fwww.reuters.com%2Farticle%2Fuk-factcheck-coronavirus-bill-gates-micr-idUSKBN21I3EC. Accessed September 17, 2022.

15. Reuters Staff. Fact check: quantum dot dye technology does not feature microchips. *Reuters.* January 6, 2022. Available at: https://www.reuters.com/article/uk-factcheck-coronavirus-bill-gates-micr-idUSKBN21I3EC. Accessed September 23, 2022.

16. Kertscher T. Biden, Harris distrusted Trump with COVID-19 vaccines, not the vaccines themselves. *Politifact.* June 23, 2021. Available at: https://www.politifact.com/factchecks/2021/jul/23/tiktok-posts/biden-harris-doubted-trump-covid-19-vaccines-not-v. Accessed August 14, 2022.

17. Yahoo News. Newsmaker plenary with former vice president Joe Biden. August 6, 2020. Available at: https://www.youtube.com/watch?v=iCpyx2T-lDA&t=863s. Accessed September 23, 2022.

18. Hamel L, Sparks G, Brodie M. KFF COVID-19 vaccine monitor: February 2021. KFF. February 26, 2021. Available at: https://www.kff.org/coronavirus-covid-19/poll-finding/kff-covid-19-vaccine-monitor-february-2021. Accessed September 23, 2022.

19. Holtzman D, Neumann M, Sumartojo E, Lansky A. Behavioral and social sciences and public health at CDC. Centers for Disease Control, MMWR. 2006;55(Suppl 2):14–16. Available at: https://www.cdc.gov/mmwr/preview/mmwrhtml/su5502a6.htm. Accessed September 23, 2022.

20. US Department of Health and Human Services. HHS launches "We Can Do This: Live" initiative to increase COVID-19 vaccine confidence. April 22, 2021. Available at: https://www.hhs.gov/about/news/2021/04/22/hhs-launches-we-can-do-this-live-initiative-increase-covid-19-vaccine-confidence.html. Accessed September 17, 2022.

21. US Department of Health and Human Services. About the campaign. COVID-19 education campaign. July 18, 2022. Available at: https://wecandothis.hhs.gov/about. Accessed September 17, 2022.

22. Adforum. AdTechCares partners with the Veterans Coalition for vaccination and Venables Bell + partners to launch Vaccine Trust PSA campaign. March 16, 2021. Available at: https://www.adforum.com/news/adtechcares-partners-with-the-veterans-coalition-for-vaccination-and-venables-bell-partners-to-launch-vaccine-trust-psa-campaign. Accessed September 23, 2022.

23. Acharya B, Dhakal C. Implementation of state vaccine incentive lottery programs and uptake of COVID-19 vaccinations in the United States. *JAMA Network Open.* 2021;4(12). doi:10.1001/jamanetworkopen.2021.38238.

24. The White House. Fact sheet: President Biden to announce goal to administer at least one vaccine shot to 70% of the US adult population by July 4th. May 4, 2021. Available at:

https://www.whitehouse.gov/briefing-room/statements-releases/2021/05/04/fact-sheet-president-biden-to-announce-goal-to-administer-at-least-one-vaccine-shot-to-70-of-the-u-s-adult-population-by-july-4th. Accessed September 23, 2022.

25. The White House. Remarks by President Biden on the COVID-19 response and the vaccination program. July 6, 2021. Available at: https://www.whitehouse.gov/briefing-room/speeches-remarks/2021/07/06/remarks-by-president-biden-on-the-covid-19-response-and-the-vaccination-program-6. Accessed September 17, 2022.

26. UNICEF. Immunization. https://www.unicef.org/immunization. Accessed September 23, 2022.

27. Toumi M, Ricciardi W. The economic value of vaccination: why prevention is wealth. *J Mark Access Health Policy*. 2015;3(2015). doi:10.3402/jmahp.v3.29414.

28. Vaccinate Your Family. Vaccines are cost saving. Updated October 19, 2020. Available at: https://vaccinateyourfamily.org/why-vaccinate/vaccine-benefits/costs-of-disease-outbreaks. Accessed September 17, 2022.

29. Association for Professionals in Infection Control and Epidemiology. Herd immunity. Updated June 6, 2021. Available at: https://apic.org/monthly_alerts/herd-immunity. Accessed September 23, 2022.

30. MacMillan C. Herd immunity: will we ever get there? *Yale Medicine*. May 21, 2021. Available at: https://www.yalemedicine.org/news/herd-immunity. Accessed September 23, 2022.

31. Bergstrom CT, Dean N. What the proponents of "natural" herd immunity don't say. *New York Times*. May 1, 2020. Available at: https://www.nytimes.com/2020/05/01/opinion/sunday/coronavirus-herd-immunity.html. Accessed September 23, 2022.

32. McNeil DG. How much herd immunity is enough? *New York Times*. December 24, 2020. Available at: https://www.nytimes.com/2020/12/24/health/herd-immunity-covid-coronavirus.html. Accessed September 23, 2022.

33. Stieg C. Dr. Fauci: "Things are going to get worse"—here's what that could look like. *Make It/CNBC*. August 5, 2021. Available at: https://www.cnbc.com/2021/08/05/dr-fauci-things-will-get-worse-amid-covid-delta-surge-unvaccinated.html. Accessed September 23, 2022.

34. Fraser MR. Harassment of health officials: a significant threat to the public's health. *Am J Public Health*. 2022;112(5):728–730. doi:10.2105/ajph.2022.306797.

35. Ward JA, Stone EM, Mui P, Resnick B. Pandemic-related workplace violence and its impact on public health officials, March 2020–January 2021. *Am J Public Health*. 2022;112(5):736–746. doi:10.2105/ajph.2021.306649.

36. Johns Hopkins University Bloomberg School of Public Health. We stand with public health: a call to action. 2021. Available at: https://standwithpublichealth.jhsph.edu. Accessed September 23, 2022.

37. Clinton, WJ. Jason Isbell: How to find something to love [Why am I telling you this? Podcast]. The Clinton Foundation. February 17, 2022. https://www.clintonfoundation.org/podcast/jason-isbell-how-to-find-something-to-love. Accessed August 14, 2022.

38. Hussain A, Ali S, Ahmed M, Hussain S. The anti-vaccination movement: a regression in modern medicine. *Cureus*. July 2018. doi:10.7759/cureus.2919.

39. College of Physicians of Philadelphia. Misconceptions about vaccines: history of anti-vaccination movements. Available at: https://historyofvaccines.org/vaccines-101/misconceptions-about-vaccines/history-anti-vaccination-movements. Accessed September 23, 2022.

40. National Conference of State Legislatures. States with religious and philosophical exemptions from school immunization requirements. May 5, 2022. Available at: https://www.ncsl.org/research/health/school-immunization-exemption-state-laws.aspx. Accessed September 23, 2022.

41. Washington State Department of Health. Measles 2019. Updated 2019. Available at: https://doh.wa.gov/you-and-your-family/illness-and-disease-z/measles/measles-2019. Accessed September 23, 2022.

42. Worden L, Ackley SF, Zipprich J, et al. Measles transmission during a large outbreak in California. *Epidemics*. 2020;30:100375. doi:10.1016/j.epidem.2019.100375.

43. Zucker JR, Rosen JB, Iwamoto M, et al. Consequences of undervaccination—measles outbreak, New York City, 2018–2019. *NEJM*. 2020;382(11):1009–1017. doi:10.1056/nejmoa1912514.

44. Hall V, Banerjee E, Kenyon C, et al. Measles Outbreak—Minnesota April–May 2017. *MMWR*. 2017;66(27):713–717.

45. Belluz J. Minnesota's measles outbreak is what happens when anti-vaxxers target immigrants. *Vox*. October 26, 2017. Available at: https://www.vox.com/science-and-health/2017/10/26/16552864/minnesotas-measles-outbreak-immigrants-anti-vaxxers. Accessed September 23, 2022.

46. Mariner WK, Annas GJ, Glantz LH. *Jacobson v. Massachusetts*: it's not your great-great-grandfather's public health law. *Am J Public Health*. 2005;95(4):581–590. doi:10.2105/ajph.2004.055160.

47. Wills M. What makes vaccine mandates legal? *JSTOR Daily*. September 3, 2021. Available at: https://daily.jstor.org/what-makes-vaccine-mandates-legal. Accessed September 23, 2022.

48. *Jacobson v. Massachusetts*, 197 US 11 (1905). *Justia Law*. February 20, 1905. Available at: https://supreme.justia.com/cases/federal/us/197/11. Accessed September 23, 2022.

49. *Jacobson v. Massachusetts*, 197 US 11 (1905). US Supreme Court. February 20, 1905. Available at: https://tile.loc.gov/storage-services/service/ll/usrep/usrep109/usrep109003/usrep109003.pdf. Accessed September 23, 2022.

50. Hotez PJ. America's deadly flirtation with antiscience and the medical freedom movement. *J Clin Invest*. February 25, 2021. Available at: https://www.jci.org/articles/view/149072. Accessed September 23, 2022.

51. Wakefield AJ, Murch SH, Anthony A, et al. Retracted: Ileal-lymphoid-nodular hyperplasia, non-specific colitis, and pervasive developmental disorder in children. *Lancet*. 1998;351(9103):637–641. doi:10.1016/s0140-6736(97)11096-0.

52. Deer B. *The Doctor Who Fooled the World: Science, Deception, and the War on Vaccines*. Baltimore, MD: Johns Hopkins University Press; 2020.

53. Institute of Medicine (US) Immunization Safety Review Committee. *Immunization Safety Review: Vaccines and Autism*. Washington, DC: National Academies Press; 2004.

54. Carlson A. Trump celebrates autism awareness day . . . after years of falsely claiming vaccines cause autism. *People*. April 2, 2019. Available at: https://people.com/politics/donald-trump-autism-awareness-day-vaccines-tweet. Accessed September 23, 2022.

55. Research!America. Americans speak out on vaccines and infectious disease. May 18, 2018. Available at: https://asm.org/ASM/media/Policy-and-Advocacy/asmrasurvey18.pdf. Accessed October 13, 2022.

56. Kottasová I. Around 1 million children in London offered polio boosters after virus is detected in sewage. *CNN*. August 10, 2022. Available at: https://www.cnn.com/2022/08/10/europe/polio-vaccine-children-london-intl/index.html. Accessed September 23, 2022.

57. Goodman B. New York adult diagnosed with polio, first US case in nearly a decade. *CNN*. July 22, 2022. Available at: https://www.cnn.com/2022/07/21/health/new-york-polio. Accessed September 23, 2022.

58. Cohen E. "Silent" spread of polio in New York drives CDC to consider additional vaccinations for some people. *CNN*. August 13, 2022. Available at: https://www.cnn.com/2022/08/11/health/polio-cdc-rockland-county/index.html. Accessed September 23, 2022.

59. US Senate Committee on Health, Education, Labor & Pensions. Vaccines save lives: what is driving preventable disease outbreaks? March 5, 2019. Available at: https://www.help.senate.gov/hearings/vaccines-save-lives-what-is-driving-preventable-disease-outbreaks. Accessed September 23, 2022.

60. Yaqub O, Castle-Clarke S, Sevdalis N, Chataway J. Attitudes to vaccination: a critical review. *Soc Sci & Med*. 2014;112:1–11. doi:10.1016/j.socscimed.2014.04.018.

61. MacDonald NE, SAGE Working Group on Vaccine Hesitancy. Vaccine hesitancy: definition, scope and determinants. *Vaccine*. 2015;33(34):4161–4164. doi:10.1016/j.vaccine.2015.04.036.

62. Hospital Management. China completes hospital for coronavirus patients. February 3, 2020. Available at: https://www.hospitalmanagement.net/news/coronavirus-first-hospital-china. Accessed September 23, 2022.

63. Assistant Secretary for Public Affairs. Biden–Harris administration releases two new reports on long COVID to support patients and further research. US Department of Health and Human Services. August 3, 2022. Available at: https://www.hhs.gov/about/news/2022/08/03/biden-harris-administration-releases-two-new-reports-long-covid-support-patients-further-research.html. Accessed September 23, 2022.

64. Editorial Board. Mr. Trump knew it was deadly and airborne. *New York Times*. September 9, 2020. Available at: https://www.nytimes.com/2020/09/09/opinion/trump-bob-woodward-coronavirus.html. Accessed September 23, 2022.

65. Woodward B. *Rage*. New York, NY: Simon & Schuster; 2020.

66. Wolfe D, Dale D. "It's going to disappear": a timeline of Trump's claims that Covid-19 will vanish. *CNN*. October 31, 2020. Available at: https://www.cnn.com/interactive/2020/10/politics/covid-disappearing-trump-comment-tracker. Accessed September 23, 2022.

67. CNN. A timeline of Trump's battle with COVID-19. Updated October 12, 2020. Available at: https://www.cnn.com/interactive/2020/10/politics/trump-covid-battle. Accessed September 23, 2022.

68. Kiviniemi MT, Orom H, Hay JL, Waters EA. Prevention is political: political party affiliation predicts perceived risk and prevention behaviors for COVID-19. *BMC Public Health*. 2022;22(1). doi:10.1186/s12889-022-12649-4.

69. Wood D, Brumfiel G. Pro-Trump counties continue to suffer far higher COVID death tolls. *NPR News*. WBUR. May 19, 2022. Available at: https://www.wbur.org/npr/1098543849/pro-trump-counties-continue-to-suffer-far-higher-covid-death-tolls. Accessed August 14, 2022.

70. Sehgal NJ, Yue D, Pope E, Wang RH, Roby D. The association between COVID-19 mortality and the county-level partisan divide in the United States. *Health Aff*. 2022;41(6). doi10.1377/hlthaff.2022.00085.

71. Miller, M. Focus group: vaccine-hesitant Republicans want facts, not emotion. de Beaumont Foundation. March 16, 2021. Available at: https://debeaumont.org/news/2021/focus-group-vaccines-republicans. Accessed September 17, 2022.

72. de Beaumont Foundation. New poll reveals most effective language to improve COVID-19 vaccine acceptance. December 2020. Available at: https://debeaumont.org/changing-the-covid-conversation/vaccineacceptance. Accessed September 23, 2022.

73. Diamond D. "We want to be educated, not indoctrinated," say Trump voters wary of coronavirus vaccination. *Washington Post.* March 15, 2021. Available at: https://www .washingtonpost.com/health/2021/03/15/vaccine-hesitant-republicans-focus-group. Accessed September 23, 2022.

74. Phillips M. "The truth is the truth": Biden's chief of staff Ron Klain doubles down on morbid White House statement saying the vaccinated have "done the right thing" and the unvaccinated are "looking at a winter of severe illness and death for you and your families." *Daily Mail Online.* December 20, 2021. Available at: https://www.dailymail.co.uk/news/article-10329217/Ron-Klain-defends-message-unvaccinated-looking-winter-severe-illness-death.html. Accessed September 23, 2022.

75. Bracken M. How the public's views on COVID-19 have shifted since the pandemic began. Morning Consult. July 27, 2022. Updated October 26, 2022. Available at: https://morningconsult .com/views-on-the-pandemic. Accessed September 17, 2022.

76. Simmons-Duffin S. CDC's new COVID metrics can leave individuals struggling to understand their risk. *Shots.* National Public Radio. March 12, 2022. Available at: https://www.npr .org/sections/health-shots. Accessed September 23, 2022.

77. Zink A. Alaska did well early in the pandemic. Then the misinformation and distrust kicked in. *Washington Post.* October 27, 2021. Available at: https://www.washingtonpost.com/opinions/2021/10/27/alaska-did-well-early-pandemic-then-misinformation-distrust-kicked. Accessed September 23, 2022.

78. Centers for Disease Control and Prevention. Vaccinate with Confidence. October 11, 2019. Available at: https://www.cdc.gov/vaccines/partners/downloads/Vaccinate-Confidently-2019 .pdf. Accessed September 23, 2022.

79. Fraser MR. Blinding me with science: complementary "head" and "heart" messages are needed to counter rising vaccine hesitancy. *J Pub Health Manage Pract.* 2019;25(5):511–514. doi:10.1097/phh.0000000000001065.

80. Sparks G, Lopes L, Montero A, et al. KFF COVID-19 Vaccine Monitor: April 2022. Kaiser Family Foundation. May 4, 2022. Available at: https://www.kff.org/coronavirus-covid-19/poll-finding/kff-covid-19-vaccine-monitor-april-2022. Accessed September 23, 2022.

81. National Medical Association. NMA COVID-19 Task Force on Vaccines and Therapeutics. Advisory statement on Federal Drug Administration's emergency use authorization approval for Pfizer and Moderna vaccine. December 21, 2020. Available at: https://www.nmanet.org/news/544970/NMA-COVID-19-Task-Force-on-Vaccines-and-Therapeutics.htm. Accessed September 23, 2022.

82. Association of State and Territorial Health Officials. Safety, not politics, must drive COVID-19 vaccine timeline. [Press release]. September 3, 2020. Available at: https://www.astho.org/

communications/newsroom/older-releases/safety-not-politics-must-drive-covid-19-vaccine-timeline. Accessed September 23, 2022.

83. Reuters Staff. Trump says without proof that FDA "deep state" slowing COVID trials. *Reuters.* August 22, 2020. Available at: https://www.reuters.com/article/us-health-coronavirus-trump-fda/trump-says-without-proof-that-fda-deep-state-slowing-covid-trials-idUSKBN25I0LF. Accessed September 23, 2022.

84. Levine D, Taylor M. Exclusive: Top FDA official says would resign if agency rubber-stamps an unproven COVID-19 vaccine. *Reuters.* August 20, 2020. Available at: https://www.reuters.com/article/us-health-coronavirus-vaccines-fda-exclu/exclusive-top-fda-official-says-would-resign-if-agency-rubber-stamps-an-unproven-covid-19-vaccine-idUSKBN25H03H. Accessed September 23, 2022.

85. Hamel L, Lopes L, Kearney A, Brodie M. KFF COVID-19 vaccine monitor: March 2021. KFF. March 30, 2021. Available at: https://www.kff.org/coronavirus-covid-19/poll-finding/kff-covid-19-vaccine-monitor-march-2021. Accessed September 23, 2022.

86. Center for Countering Digital Hate. Anti-vaxx misinformation. [Blog]. Available at: https://counterhate.com/topic/anti-vaxx-misinformation. Accessed September 23, 2022.

87. Center for Countering Digital Hate. Substack & anti-vaxx newsletters. Available at: https://counterhate.com/research/substack-anti-vaxx-newsletters. Accessed September 23, 2022.

88. Pandemic profiteers: the business of anti-vaxx. Center for Countering Digital Hate. Posted June 1, 2021. Available at: https://twitter.com/reportbywilson/status/1552322518857293824. Accessed August 14, 2022.

89. Haileyesus S. How to make money on social media. *Small Business Trends.* March 18, 2022. Available at: https://smallbiztrends.com/2021/09/how-to-make-money-on-social-media.html. Accessed September 23, 2022.

90. de Beaumont Foundation. The dangerous link between social media, misinformation, and vaccination rates. November 4, 2021. Available at: https://debeaumont.org/wp-content/uploads/2021/11/SociaMediaPoll-1.pdf. Accessed September 23, 2022.

91. de Beaumont Foundation. Study: Americans who get COVID-19 information from social media more likely to believe misinformation, less likely to be vaccinated. November 4, 2021. Available at: https://debeaumont.org/news/2021/social-media-misinformation-poll. Accessed September 23, 2022.

92. Center for Countering Digital Hate. The anti-vaxx playbook. 2020. Available at: https://counterhate.com/wp-content/uploads/2022/05/210106-The-Anti-Vaxx-Playbook.pdf. Accessed September 23, 2022.

93. Greenberg J. Donald Trump's false claim that doctors inflate COVID-19 deaths to make more money. *Politifact.* November 1, 2020. Available at: https://www.politifact.com/factchecks/2020/nov/01/donald-trump/donald-trumps-false-claim-doctors-inflate-covid-19. Accessed September 23, 2022.

94. Hotez PJ. 2021. Mounting antiscience aggression in the United States. *PLOS Biol.* 19(7). doi:10.1371/journal.pbio.3001369.

95. Hotez PJ. 2021. Anti-science kills: from Soviet embrace of pseudoscience to accelerated attacks on US biomedicine. *PLOS Biol.* 19(1):e3001068. Available at: https://doi.org/10.1371/journal.pbio.3001068. Accessed September 23, 2022.

96. Hotez P. Covid vaccines: Time to confront anti-vax aggression. *Nature*. April 27, 2021. Available at: https://www.nature.com/articles/d41586-021-01084-x. Accessed September 23, 2022.

97. Hotez PJ. The antiscience movement is escalating, going global and killing thousands. *Scientific American*. March 29, 2021. Available at: https://www.scientificamerican.com/article/the-antiscience-movement-is-escalating-going-global-and-killing-thousands. Accessed September 23, 2022.

98. Quote Investigator. A lie can travel halfway around the world while the truth is putting on its shoes. July 13, 2014. Last updated November 6, 2017. Available at: https://quoteinvestigator.com/2014/07/13/truth. Accessed September 17, 2022.

99. Swift J. A quote by Jonathan Swift. Goodreads. Available at: https://www.goodreads.com/quotes/7649282-falsehood-flies-and-truth-comes-limping-after-it-so-that. Accessed September 17, 2022.

100. Thucydides. A quote from Thucydides, *History of the Peloponnesian War*. Goodreads. Available at: https://www.goodreads.com/quotes/336570-most-people-in-fact-will-not-take-the-trouble-in. Accessed September 17, 2022.

101. Washington HA. *Medical Apartheid: The Dark History of Medical Experimentation on Black Americans from Colonial Times to the Present*. New York, NY: Doubleday; 2006.

102. McVean A. 40 years of human experimentation in America: the Tuskegee study. Office for Science and Society, McGill University. January 25, 2019. Available at: https://www.mcgill.ca/oss/article/history/40-years-human-experimentation-america-tuskegee-study. Accessed September 23, 2022.

103. Jones JH. *Bad Blood: The Tuskegee Syphilis Experiment*. New York, NY: Free Press; 1993.

104. Manning, KD. More than medical mistrust. *The Lancet*. 2020;396(10261):1481–1482. Available at: https://doi.org/10.1016/s0140-6736(20)32286-8. Accessed September 17, 2022.

105. Siegel M, Critchfield-Jain I, Boykin M, et al. Racial/ethnic disparities in state-level COVID-19 vaccination rates and their association with structural racism. *J Racial Ethnic Health Disparities*. October 2021. doi:10.1007/s40615-021-01173-7.

106. Norris ML. Black people are justifiably wary of a vaccine. Their trust must be earned. *The Washington Post*. December 9, 2020. Available at: https://www.washingtonpost.com/opinions/black-people-are-justifiably-wary-of-a-vaccine-their-trust-must-be-earned/2020/12/09/4cf5f18c-3a36-11eb-9276-ae0ca72729be_story.html. Accessed September 23, 2022.

107. American Medical Association. What is structural racism? Updated November 9, 2021. Available at: https://www.ama-assn.org/delivering-care/health-equity/what-structural-racism. Accessed September 23, 2022.

108. Padamsee TJ, Bond RM, Dixon GN, et al. Changes in COVID-19 vaccine hesitancy among Black and white individuals in the US. *JAMA Network Open*. 2022;5(1). doi:10.1001/jamanetworkopen.2021.44470.

109. Bollyky TJ, Hulland EN, Barber RM, et al. Pandemic preparedness and COVID-19: an exploratory analysis of infection and fatality rates, and contextual factors associated with preparedness in 177 countries, from Jan 1, 2020, to Sept 30, 2021. *The Lancet*. 2022;399(10334):1489–1512. doi:10.1016/s0140-6736(22)00172-6.

110. Association of State and Territorial Health Officers. Enhancing trust in public health: when recommendations change. Available at: https://www.astho.org/globalassets/pdf/covid/

enhancing-trust-in-public-health-when-recommendations-change.pdf. Accessed: September 23, 2022.

111. Harvard T.H. Chan School of Public Health. The public's perspective on the United States public health system. Robert Wood Johnson Foundation and Harvard School of Public Health. May 13, 2021. Available at: https://www.rwjf.org/en/library/research/2021/05/the-publics-perspective-on-the-united-states-public-health-system.html. Accessed September 23, 2022.

112. Bellis MA, Hughes K, Ford K, et al. Associations between adverse childhood experiences, attitudes towards COVID-19 restrictions and vaccine hesitancy: a cross-sectional study. *BMJ Open*. 2022;12(2):1–10. doi:10.1136/bmjopen-2021-053915.

113. Klein E. The COVID policy that really mattered wasn't a policy. *New York Times*. February 6, 2022. Available at: https://www.nytimes.com/2022/02/06/opinion/covid-pandemic-policy-trust.html. Accessed September 23, 2022.

8

A Fair Shot

The attitude here is the oxygen mask approach. We want to get our oxygen mask on first and then we're going to help the people around us.[1]

-Operation Warp Speed official, May 12, 2020

Vaccinating all the world at once has never been done. But if we can put a rover on Mars, we can surely produce billions of vaccines and save lives on earth.[2]

-Dr. Tedros Adhanom Ghebreyesus, Director General,
World Health Organization, March 5, 2021

Vaccine nationalism is ethically inexcusable but politically inevitable. Must increase production.[3]

-Dr. Tom Frieden, March 27, 2022

As we finalize this manuscript in the summer of 2022, over 12 billion doses of COVID vaccine have been administered in 184 countries across the globe.[4] America, the envy of the world in early 2021 when it owned a disproportionate supply of vaccines, was near the top of all nations in vaccination rates in early 2021. But by midsummer we had lost our lead. By August 2022, the United States had fallen to 52nd place in the world, between Sri Lanka and Fiji, on the percentage of individuals who have received one dose of a COVID vaccine.[5] While the story of how vaccine hesitancy and a lack of confidence in COVID vaccines contributed to how we lost this lead in America, another important question is, Despite lagging rates in our country, what has America done to help vaccinate the world? This chapter briefly examines what it will take to give everyone on the planet a fair shot at being vaccinated against COVID.

Viruses know no national borders. In our ever increasingly global world, individuals can travel from any side of the globe to another in less than 24 hours, carrying with them a novel pathogen that can ignite a global pandemic. Efforts to pin blame on a country or a region for the emergence of such threats may make politicians and their followers feel better but do nothing to interrupt viral transmission between people in our tightly connected world. Travel bans and country lockdowns can often tame the spread of a disease, but, as we saw with COVID, ultimately do little to truly stop it. COVID's global impact reminds us of just how fast, and just how deadly, the spread of a new pathogen can be even with the best of international cooperation and coordinated efforts to stop it.

A slogan adopted by the Global Vaccine Alliance, or Gavi, states that "no one is safe until everyone is safe."[6] Dr. Seth Berkley, an American epidemiologist who leads Gavi, expanded on that theme in an October 2021 communique to the leaders of the G20 countries. "Failing to get more vaccines to people in all countries more quickly—is the principal reason why the virus is still winning," Dr. Berkley told the leaders of the world's 20 biggest economies.[7] He continued:

> Until now governments have focused on tackling the pandemic at the national level, striving to achieve high vaccination coverage within their own borders, rather than building it up globally. This has only prolonged the pandemic. But with infectious disease you cannot extinguish a global inferno one country at a time. It needs to be simultaneously stamped out all across the world, or it will just continue to spread, increasing the risk of new and potentially more dangerous variants emerging.[7]

The stakes could not be stated more clearly. Dr. Tedros Adhanom Ghebreyesus, director general of the World Health Organization (WHO), made a similar point in March 2021 when he urged the world to grab the opportunity to get everyone vaccinated "with both hands." Pointing out that failure to vaccinate and prevent COVID transmission in every country would not only promote needless suffering but also contribute to viral evolution and immune escape, he writes:

> Any opportunity to beat this virus should be grabbed with both hands. New variants are appearing that show signs of being more transmissible, more deadly and less susceptible to vaccines. The threat is clear: as long as the virus is spreading anywhere, it has more opportunities to mutate and potentially undermine the efficacy of vaccines everywhere. We could end up back at square one.[2]

And given the toll COVID has taken worldwide over the last two and a half years, getting back to "square one" should be avoided at all costs.

Gavi, an international nongovernmental organization based in Geneva, Switzerland, is the only organization with the capacity to pull together the key players necessary to conduct a global COVID vaccination campaign. The organization has worked to increase sustainable and equitable vaccination in the world's poorest countries since 2000. The list of key stakeholders is long and includes the WHO, UNICEF, the World Bank, the Bill & Melinda Gates Foundation, and other donors, among them sovereign governments, private-sector foundations and corporate partners, nongovernmental organizations, advocacy groups, professional and community associations, faith-based organizations, and academia. It also includes vaccine manufacturers, among them those in emerging markets and in research and technical health institutes. Much like the vaccination campaign in every US jurisdiction, the effort to vaccinate everyone cannot succeed without extensive partnership and coordination. Nor can it succeed without an understanding of the collective risk diseases pose to the entire globe.

Gavi's role in leading this global vaccine campaign was set early in the pandemic. The WHO, anticipating that providing fair and equitable access to tools needed to fight COVID across the globe would be an enormous challenge, hosted a gathering in April 2020 to launch the Access to COVID-19 Tools (ACT) Accelerator. The initiative brought together governments, scientific and regulatory experts, philanthropies, and global health organizations to focus on four main pillars: diagnostics, treatment, vaccines, and health systems strengthening. Each of the pillars is led and coordinated by different multilateral institutions. COVAX, the COVID-19 Vaccines Global Access, is coled by the Coalition for Epidemic Preparedness Innovations, Gavi, and the WHO, with a focus on the vaccine pillar of the ACT Accelerator. The goal of the effort is to quicken the development and production of COVID-19 vaccines and to guarantee fair and equitable access for every country in the world.[8]

Mirroring some of the development elements of Operation Warp Speed, this global mechanism was envisioned to "act as a platform that will support the research, development and manufacturing of a wide range of COVID-19 vaccine candidates, and negotiate their pricing."[8]

The original COVAX plan was for all participating countries, regardless of income levels, to have equal access to vaccines once developed. The aim was to have two billion doses available by the end of 2021, which was predicted to be enough to protect high-risk and vulnerable people, as well as frontline health care workers. *STAT News* summarized the effort as follows:

> It would be an end-to-end program—spanning vaccine development to delivery—for every country in the world. By investing in several vaccine candidates from different companies, COVAX would improve its chances of having a successful vaccine when trials concluded. Buying doses in bulk would mean COVAX could negotiate favorable prices with manufacturers. High- and middle-income countries would buy into COVAX, while poorer ones would receive vaccines for free, funded by donations from wealthy governments and charities, for up to 20% of their population. As a clearing house, COVAX would allocate vaccines fairly across the globe, shipping them to rich and poor countries simultaneously. Such a system could be established fairly straightforwardly, the proposal said, with sufficient political will and public sector financing.[9]

But much like the bumpy vaccine roll out in the United States, the global plan soon faced challenges. Most significantly, the Trump administration, on the heels of withdrawing from WHO in July 2020, declined to join the effort. The Trump White House rationale was clear: "The United States will continue to engage our international partners to ensure we defeat this virus, but we will not be constrained by multilateral organizations influenced by the corrupt World Health Organization and China," stated the White House spokesperson.[10] The decision seemed to contradict a much more promising statement on global vaccine diplomacy shared by the president just two months earlier at the May 15, 2020, White House launch of Operation Warp Speed. At that time, he stated, "We're also working very strongly with other countries who are also—have some great, great scientists, doctors. And we're all working very closely together, and they're viewing us as the leader, and we are—the relationship with other countries on solving this problem has been incredible."[11]

Despite the abrupt shift in policy, on January 16, 2021, just one year and one week after the virus genome was sequenced, COVAX began delivering doses to the world. The first COVAX vaccine reached Africa on March 1, 2021. As in the United States and elsewhere, to get vaccines rolling health authorities had to overcome a thousand logistical challenges, including cold chain requirements, rampant misinformation, and pockets of hesitation. But more than anything, the biggest barrier to COVAX's work was vaccine supply. When COVAX doses first reached Africa, the director general of WHO, Dr. Tedros Adhanom Ghebreyesus, stated, "This was undoubtedly a moment of celebration that the miracle of science was being shared—but it was offset by the shame that many countries hit hard during the pandemic have still not received any vaccines."[2]

Amid nearly daily warnings from the WHO and others about widening global vaccine inequity between high- and low-resource countries, a major blow to the COVAX effort came when the COVID Delta variant quickly spread through India in the spring of 2021. COVAX relies heavily on Indian vaccine manufacturers, but given the conditions in India those manufacturers imposed a de facto export ban, which crippled the ability of COVAX to meet its aspirations.[12] By September 2021, COVAX had delivered only 250 million doses to participating countries, far below its projections—and just as in the United States critics pounced, calling the COVAX effort "naively ambitious" and worse.[9] In response, again just as in the United States, the leaders at COVAX responded with creativity and persistence.

The United States rejoined WHO under the Biden administration and in February 2021 reestablished its global leadership position by committing $4 billion to the COVAX effort.[13] The United States also announced a series of vaccine donations and in September 2021 announced the purchase of 500 million Pfizer doses to donate to the COVAX effort. As welcome as the donations were in the short term, several international health groups, including Doctors Without Borders, pointed out the shortcomings of any donation strategy that relies solely on the goodwill of donor nations. In September 2021, the group reported, "The vast majority of lofty donation pledges haven't materialized so far; only 15 percent of the more than 1 billion doses pledged by wealthy governments have arrived in Africa."[14]

It was clear that the "America First" advance vaccine purchase policies initiated under the Trump administration and continued in large part by President Biden in effect constrained supply for many vulnerable nations.[15] Unfortunately, the United States was not alone among high-resource countries in establishing such policies.

The global criticism of wealthy nations cornering the supply on vaccine was further amplified by state strategies to vaccinate any willing and eligible patient, even if that meant puncturing a full vial of vaccine just to use one dose and discarding the rest 12 hours later when it expired.[16] The wastage policy, which may have been successful in promoting vaccination domestically, created vigorous debate among state health leaders who understood the urgency of getting all Americans vaccinated but also emphasized global equity in response to COVID burden overseas. Ultimately, an estimated 82 million doses of vaccine were wasted in the United States between December 2020 and May 2022 as a result of the need to destroy expired vaccine, vials that were unusable because they were not properly stored at required temperatures, and partially used vaccine vials that required destruction after being open beyond the time allowed.[17]

The "me first" attitude of many nations when it came to vaccines was dubbed vaccine nationalism, an attitude that characterized many high-income nations.[18] These policies came under withering criticism. As Dr. Tom Frieden noted in the tweet quoted earlier, vaccine nationalism is both inexcusable and inevitable.[3] It also put COVAX in the impossible position of having to condemn the very countries it relied on for both funding and eventual vaccine donations. Future responses should encourage global cooperation, not shun it, especially when medical countermeasures become available.

To address the issue, many global health advocates demanded that both Pfizer and Moderna share their technology to allow others to begin local manufacturing, especially in Africa. South Africa and India put forth a proposal to the World Trade Organization to make an emergency waiver of intellectual property rights to facilitate more widespread vaccine manufacturing. The proposal was supported by over 100 countries. Even the United States announced support on May 5, 2021, stating that despite long-standing support for intellectual property protections, the extraordinary circumstances of a global pandemic required extraordinary measures.[19] However, more than a year later, as this book goes to press no action has been taken.

Despite these roadblocks, by January 15, 2022, COVAX had shipped one billion doses of COVID vaccine to countries worldwide.[20] Reflecting on the achievement, global health leader Richard Hatchett said, "People [believe] COVAX has been a terrible failure because it didn't hit the two billion dose target. And it didn't, and we're disappointed," he told *STAT News*.[21] "But delivering a billion doses in 13 months relative to any historic example or any comparable experience with trying to move new medical products to create global equity—that's clearly unprecedented." By the end of May 2022, that number had climbed to 1.5 billion doses, with 500 million of those delivered to Africa.[22]

A VIRUS ANYWHERE IS JUST A PLANE RIDE AWAY

There is a long road ahead, but the global success to date should also be celebrated. In a modeling study by Imperial College in London released in June 2022, researchers estimated that globally vaccinations prevented 14.4 million deaths from COVID-19 in 185 countries between December 8, 2020, and December 8, 2021.[23] This estimate rose to 19.8 million deaths from COVID-19 averted when they used excess deaths as an estimate of the true extent of the pandemic, representing a global reduction of 63% in total deaths during just the first year of COVID-19 vaccination efforts. Furthermore, they estimated that in the COVAX Advance Market Commitment countries 41% of excess mortality was averted (7.4 million of 17.9 million deaths). Finally, they estimated that in low-income countries an additional 45% of deaths could have been averted had the 20% vaccination coverage target set by COVAX been met by each country and that an additional 111% of deaths could have been averted had the 40% target set by WHO been met by each country by the end of 2021. The researchers concluded the study by stating, "COVID-19 vaccination has substantially altered the course of the pandemic, saving tens of millions of lives globally. However, inadequate access to vaccines in low-income countries has limited the impact in these settings, reinforcing the need for global vaccine equity and coverage."[23]

Dr. Frieden often incorporated the statement "A virus anywhere is just a plane ride away" into most of his public comments, most prominently in a September 10, 2013, address to the National Press Club about a year before the United States had its first encounter with Ebola on its shores.[24] He and several others have for years been urging American leaders to acknowledge that in an interconnected world, investments in protecting our health require as much prioritization as investments in the nation's military defense. A traveler arriving in the United States most likely brought the first case of COVID to the country from overseas in January 2020. It did not take a great deal of premonition to predict the results of underinvestment and underpreparedness in global public health when that plane arrived. Clearly, when it comes to infectious diseases, global action matters. While it appears America is on the right track in support of global efforts to promote COVID vaccination, much work remains to be done to counter vaccine nationalism if we are to achieve a fair shot for everyone.

REFERENCES

1. Cohen J. Unveiling "Warp Speed," the White House's America-first push for a coronavirus vaccine. *Science*. May 12, 2020. Available at: https://www.science.org/content/article/unveiling-warp-speed-white-house-s-america-first-push-coronavirus-vaccine. Accessed September 20, 2022.

2. Ghebreyesus TA. A "me first" approach to vaccination won't defeat Covid. *Guardian*. March 5, 2021. Available at: https://www.theguardian.com/commentisfree/2021/mar/05/vaccination-covid-vaccines-rich-nations. Accessed September 20, 2022.

3. Frieden T (@DrTomFrieden). Vaccine nationalism is ethically inexcusable but politically inevitable. Must increase production. Twitter. Posted March 26, 2021. Available at: https://mobile.twitter.com/DrTomFrieden/status/1375999574442708992. Accessed September 23, 2022.

4. Randall T, Sam C, Tartar A, et al. More than 12.4 billion shots given: Covid-19 tracker. *Bloomberg.com*. Updated September 20, 2022. Available at: https://www.bloomberg.com/graphics/covid-vaccine-tracker-global-distribution. Accessed September 23, 2022.

5. Holder J. Tracking coronavirus vaccinations around the world. *New York Times*. January 29, 2021. Updated September 4, 2022. Available at: https://www.nytimes.com/interactive/2021/world/covid-vaccinations-tracker.html. Accessed September 20, 2022.

6. Berkley S. No one is safe until everyone is safe. Gavi, the Vaccine Alliance. October 29, 2021. Available at: https://www.gavi.org/vaccineswork/no-one-safe-until-everyone-safe. Accessed September 20, 2022.

7. Berkley S. G20 Italy, the Rome Summit. PageSuite. Available at: https://edition.pagesuite-professional.co.uk/html5/reader/production/default.aspx?pubname=&edid=5bf5bf93-2829-43df-a51e-35ef37ce39dd. Accessed September 23, 2022.

8. Gavi, the Vaccine Alliance. What is COVAX? Available at: https://www.gavi.org/covax-facility#what. Accessed September 20, 2022.

9. Goldhill O. "Naively ambitious": how COVAX failed on its promise to vaccinate the world. *STAT*. October 8, 2021. Available at: https://www.statnews.com/2021/10/08/how-covax-failed-on-its-promise-to-vaccinate-the-world. Accessed September 20, 2022.

10. Rauhala E, Abutaleb Y. US says it won't join WHO-linked effort to develop, distribute coronavirus vaccine. *Washington Post*. September 1, 2020. Available at: https://www.washingtonpost.com/world/coronavirus-vaccine-trump/2020/09/01/b44b42be-e965-11ea-bf44-0d31c85838a5_story.html. Accessed September 20, 2022.

11. National Archives and Records Administration. Remarks by President Trump on vaccine development. May 15, 2020. Available at: https://trumpwhitehouse.archives.gov/briefings-statements/remarks-president-trump-vaccine-development. Accessed September 20, 2022.

12. Findlay S, Peel M, Mancini DP. India blocks vaccine exports in blow to dozens of nations. *Financial Times*. March 25, 2021. Available at: https://www.ft.com/content/5349389c-8313-41e0-9a67-58274e24a019. Accessed September 20, 2022.

13. The White House. Fact sheet: President Biden to take action on global health through support of COVAX and calling for health security financing. February 18, 2021. Available at: https://www.whitehouse.gov/briefing-room/statements-releases/2021/02/18/fact-sheet-president-biden-to-take-action-on-global-health-through-support-of-covax-and-calling-for-health-security-financing. Accessed September 20, 2022.

14. Doctors Without Borders USA. US COVID-19 vaccine donations are not enough to end the pandemic. September 22, 2021. Available at: https://www.doctorswithoutborders.org/latest/us-covid-19-vaccine-donations-are-not-enough-end-pandemic. Accessed September 20, 2022.

15. Banco E. How Trump's "America first" edict delayed the global Covid fight. *Politico*. December 1, 2021. Available at: https://www.politico.com/news/2021/12/01/trump-america-first-covid-523604. Accessed September 20, 2022.

16. Centers for Disease Control and Prevention. Administration of Pfizer-BioNTech COVID-19 vaccines. June 22, 2022. Available at: https://www.cdc.gov/vaccines/covid-19/info-by-product/pfizer/administration.html. Accessed September 20, 2022.

17. Crist C. More than 82 million COVID vaccine doses wasted in US: report. WebMD. June 7, 2022. Available at: https://www.webmd.com/vaccines/covid-19-vaccine/news/20220607/millions-covid-vaccine-doses-wasted-us-report. Accessed September 20, 2022.

18. Ravelo JL. Tedros calls out "me-first" approach to COVID-19 vaccines: "this is wrong." *Devex*. January 18, 2021. Available at: https://www.devex.com/news/tedros-calls-out-me-first-approach-to-covid-19-vaccines-this-is-wrong-98937. Accessed September 24, 2022.

19. Tai K (@AmbassadorTai). These extraordinary times and circumstances call for extraordinary measures. The US supports the waiver of IP protections on COVID-19 vaccines to help end the pandemic and we'll actively participate in @WTO negotiations to make that happen. pic.twitter.com/96ERlboZS8. Twitter. Posted May 5, 2021. Available at: https://twitter.com/AmbassadorTai/status/1390021205974003720. Accessed September 20, 2022.

20. Berkley S (@GaviSeth). Proud moment in this ongoing @Gavi Board meeting when we reflected on #COVAX's key achievements over the last two years. There is still a long road ahead, but significant progress has been made in the largest and most complex global vaccine roll-out in history. #vaccineequity pic.twitter.com/fyn7nbzdyb. Twitter. Posted June 23, 2022. Available at: https://twitter.com/GaviSeth/status/1539919470612942849. Accessed September 20, 2022.

21. Branswell H. Why Covid-19 vaccines are a freaking miracle. *STAT*. February 14, 2022. https://www.statnews.com/2022/02/14/why-covid-19-vaccines-are-a-freaking-miracle. Accessed September 23, 2022.

22. Gavi, the Vaccine Alliance. COVAX deliveries. Available at: https://www.gavi.org/covax-facility. Accessed September 20, 2022.

23. Watson OJ, Barnsley G, Toor J, et al. Global impact of the first year of COVID-19 vaccination: a mathematical modelling study. *Lancet Infect Dis*. 2022;22(9):1293–1302. doi:10.1016/s1473-3099(22)00320-6.

24. Overman S. CDC director catalogs health threats that are "just a plane ride away." National Press Club. September 10, 2013. Available at: https://www.press.org/newsroom/cdc-director-catalogs-health-threats-are-just-plane-ride-away. Accessed September 20, 2022.

9

What Matters Most

So the final lesson of 1918, a simple one yet most difficult to execute, is that those who occupy positions of authority must lessen the panic that can alienate all within a society. Society cannot function if it is every man for himself. By definition, civilization cannot survive that . . . Those in authority must retain the public's trust. The way to do that is to distort nothing, to put the best face on nothing, to try to manipulate no one.[1]

–John Barry, Afterword, *The Great Influenza*

In the first year of the COVID vaccine distribution campaign in the United States, governmental public agencies oversaw the administration of close to 500 million doses of vaccine—a vaccine that was not even imagined in the year prior.[2] Numerous books and articles have been written about the scientific sprint to develop COVID vaccines and to assure their delivery nationwide. Those recountings, as important as they are to science and vaccine discovery, have never fully described what it took to take these miracle vaccines and turn them into lifesaving vaccinations. Our story focuses on the last mile, what happens in the handoff from shipment to clinic, and the last inch, that almost sacred space between a needle and an arm.

We believe that the story of the race to vaccinate America is as compelling as the world's effort to develop a COVID vaccine. We also believe that while there are many, many heroes in the COVID story, a special spot for our nation's public health professionals is well earned. In addition to the remarkable feat of supporting efforts to vaccinate large numbers of Americans, public health authorities deserve credit for many remarkable wins. For example, among the most vulnerable, the Centers for Disease Control and Prevention (CDC) estimated that close to 95% of Americans age 65 and older received at least one shot.[2] As of August 2022, the number of doses administered is approaching 600 million, with 221 million Americans fully vaccinated and over 100 million people receiving at least one booster dose providing added protection.[2]

As a result of the work of public health agencies and their partners in community-based organizations, the faith community, health care systems, community clinics, and the pharmacy sector, the inequity between white and Black Americans, at least on COVID vaccination rates, has narrowed, though equity remains a pressing problem.[3] Hispanic Americans have a vaccination rate that has surpassed that of white Americans.[3] Efforts to close the rural and urban vaccination gap continue, but thanks to dedicated public health leadership and new investments in public health infrastructure nationwide, the opportunity to close that gap is as real as ever. What public health leaders and their partners were able to do is akin to putting a person on the moon, but with an impact affecting hundreds of millions of lives. It is indeed unprecedented.

Claire Hannan highlights the extraordinary role of public health workers in her assessment of the COVID response:

> What was incredible is that the people in public health didn't buckle. They just kept going and, even though they were getting screamed at and having media articles written about their systems shutting down, you know, they just kept making adjustments . . . It was never a part of the plan for public health to vaccinate high volumes of people. And, you know, that's what they stood up and did. And it was incredible. (author oral interview with Claire Hannan, MPH, March 17, 2022)

Public health's response to COVID was not perfect. There were certainly missteps and miscalculations. Tension, conflict, and misunderstanding between public health agencies at all levels of government and between public health agencies and many other stakeholders created frustration and anger. Delays, contradictions, and changes in vaccination administration planning and communication eroded the confidence of many and in some cases ended careers. As historic as the vaccine campaign is, it was marked by challenges. The limited supply of vaccine, the late arrival of resources to fund the campaign in the early months, an election year and political upheaval just after, and persistent and pervasive vaccine hesitancy and refusal were just a few. As Dr. Marcus Plescia, chief medical officer for the Association of State and Territorial Health Officials (ASTHO), told Shepard Smith during a December 1, 2020, CNBC interview two weeks before vaccine rollout, "It's not going to be seamless, but we'll make it happen."[4]

Given the underresourced condition of state and local public health agencies prior to COVID, many of their disease surveillance systems had to be updated, duplicated, or recreated because of the need to urgently respond to a new threat. Data systems in hospitals, laboratories, and inventory management systems had to be rejiggered to meet the requirements of COVID and were constantly being updated and revised. Despite the pre-COVID establishment of an effective and functional childhood immunization system nationwide, no similarly robust system existed to support adult immunizations. That meant public health professionals and private-sector partners were essentially building such systems on the fly. Dr. Walt Orenstein, a 26-year veteran of the CDC's immunization program and a renowned expert of what it takes to turn a vaccine into a vaccination, notes, "It is amazing what was done. Despite the lack of a better functioning adult immunization structure, vaccine still got out rapidly. If we had a system where we could get 80% or 90% influenza [vaccine out] every year, then getting a new vaccine out would be a lot easier" (author oral interview with Walter A. Orenstein, MD, February 21, 2022).

Years of experience working across public and private sectors to deliver and administer routine childhood and adult vaccines, the speedy adoption of a learning-by-doing mentality, and the application of rapid quality improvement techniques—all expanded the capacity of the vaccine campaign to achieve a cadence of nearly three million shots per day in just three months. This translated to an astounding rate of more than 2,000 doses per minute at the national level. In almost every instance, public health leaders' ingenuity, creativity, and commitment to their mission helped them rise to the occasion and deliver lifesaving results.

The success of the effort came at an extraordinary cost to the mental health and well-being of public health workers, however. The near-constant pace of work and the thousand details involved in vaccinating America took a serious toll on the public health workforce, just as it has the hard work of health professionals in pharmacies, intensive care units, and clinics. As the nation was pushing to meet the president's Fourth of July goal, the CDC released results of a study showing that among public health professionals responding to COVID, 53% reported symptoms of at least one mental health condition in the preceding two weeks, including depression (32%), anxiety (30.3%), PTSD (36.8%), or suicidal ideation (8.4%).[5] Public health workers who reported being unable to take time off from work were more likely to report adverse mental health symptoms; among those not able to take time off from work, the most common reasons were concern about falling behind on work (64.4%), no work coverage (60.6%), and feeling guilty (59.0%).[5] These findings spurred new attention to building the resilience of the public health workforce and launched many state and national initiatives to address public health worker stress and burnout.[6,7] They also helped galvanize federal support for historic investments in public health workforce expansions and training programs sorely needed for years.

The Commonwealth Fund estimated that through March 2022, COVID-19 vaccination efforts in the United States prevented over 2 million deaths and 17 million hospitalizations.[8] According to the Commonwealth Fund's modeling, in the absence of vaccination we would have seen an estimated 66 million additional infections and nearly $900 billion in associated health care costs. These results have been achieved with a public taxpayer investment of less than $40 billion, with approximately $7 billion of that dedicated to vaccine distribution activities.[9]

While immense credit goes to the role the National Institutes of Health has played in basic research; the pharmaceutical industry's scientific brilliance and dedication; the military's galvanization of manufacturing, procurement, and logistics expertise; and the rapid mobilization of the clinical and pharmacy sectors, we believe the underappreciated story is how the governmental public health system at the federal, state, territorial, tribal, and local levels is largely responsible for getting so many shots in so many arms in so little time.

COVID is not going away, at least not any time soon. The world has witnessed viral evolution in real time, watching new variants emerge and take hold as earlier variants die out. Vaccines developed to stop COVID in 2020 are not as effective in stopping new COVID variants in 2022. Work is underway now to administer new bivalent vaccines to address emerging variants as COVID continues to spread, mutate, and reinfect the world. The COVID endgame is uncertain but almost certainly will rely on new vaccine formulations and increased vaccine uptake in the United States and around the world.

In January 2022, Dr. Sylvie Briand, director of the Epidemic and Pandemic Preparedness and Prevention Department at the World Health Organization, laid out three possible scenarios to help plan for what COVID may do in the future:

> Scenario 1: The virus evolves, it remains highly contagious but causes mild illness in the majority of cases. The virus can be grouped with the 4 other coronaviruses that circulate endemically. This scenario is not unrealistic, but it may take many years to be realized.

> Scenario 2: The virus continues to evolve and produces new variants. The disease presents itself as seasonal epidemics when the conditions of transmission are favorable. Since the population has basic immunity, severe forms of the disease can still be observed especially in people at risk. This scenario is similar to seasonal influenza. It will be important to continue to vaccinate at-risk groups and adopt preventive measures when transmission is high.

> Scenario 3: A new variant emerges evading acquired immunity and resulting in a large number of cases. The health system is overloaded and therefore there are more deaths. The situation is very similar to what was experienced at the beginning of 2020 in many regions of the world.[10]

Briand concludes, "We can imagine more scenarios. What matters is to plan for interventions to be ready for each of them. It is wise to hope for the best but prepare for the worst."[10] All three scenarios are plausible, and none is desirable, but these scenarios acknowledge the basic truth that regardless of what happens with COVID, it is probably with us for the long term.

Given our current situation, scenario 2 seems the most likely, but this virus has surprised us before. As such, developing and administering effective medical countermeasures, including vaccines, is a must. Developing the trust and social cohesion to support future vaccine confidence is essential. Critical to both is taking the lessons learned from our experience of the last two and a half years and applying them to our future preparedness efforts.

LESSONS LEARNED: WHAT MATTERS MOST

In October 2021, retired health care executive Ren Davis published an essay in the *Atlanta Constitution Journal* pointing out that a visit to any older cemeteries in America "illustrate[s] the tragic deaths of children (and adults) from acute infectious diseases in the 19th and early 20th centuries when vaccines to combat these scourges had not yet been developed."[11] Describing a local cemetery where he volunteers, he noted that "nearly 30% of the interments at Oakland—which was established in 1850—are children. Many died from diphtheria, typhoid fever, tetanus, pertussis (whooping cough) and other acute illnesses. These graves are a heartbreaking testament to the fragility of life in that era."[11] They are also a reminder of how far we have come in ending the scourge of many once-common preventable illnesses and death with modern vaccines.

Today, there are over one million new graves in America marking the victims of the COVID pandemic, close to half of which came after vaccines were widely available. It is impossible to know how future generations will judge a society that tolerated so many preventable deaths when a free, safe, and effective vaccine was available in abundance. Those markers testify not only to the fragility of life but also to the limits of our imagination in reaching the people who needed us most. They are stark reminders that infectious diseases are still deadly and that vaccines do not save lives, only vaccinations do. These are lessons we hope future generations do not have to relearn; they are lessons written in stone.

To date there has been no formal review or national "after action" review between state and federal public health officials to share their observations about the strengths, weaknesses, opportunities, and challenges of the two-and-half-year battle that has been COVID. While individual agencies and public health stakeholders have discussed COVID response challenges, a structured and systematic process to identify improvements and enhancements to preparedness for future pandemics has not officially taken place. No national commission has been chartered by Congress to assess what worked and what went wrong. Critically important, observations and learnings that were part of the largest public health vaccination campaign in US history and could help shape future federal, state, and local relations remain uncatalogued as a result.

As we complete this manuscript in August 2022, the World Health Organization has just declared monkeypox a public health emergency of international concern,[12] while the US secretary of health and human services has declared monkeypox a national public health emergency.[13] Public health officials are again ramping up for yet another massive vaccination campaign requiring tremendous state and federal partnership without the benefit of robust discussions about what we experienced together over the last two years. As a result, we are already seeing in the monkeypox response the same communication and coordination challenges that confounded the COVID vaccine rollout. Reinventing vaccine distribution channels; limited vaccine supply; lack of resources to promote vaccination outreach and education; data collection, sharing, and reporting issues—these are all present-day concerns that state public health leaders share with federal partners and policymakers, issues constraining the response to another vaccine-preventable disease threat.

FIVE KEY LESSONS

We offer the following five lessons in the spirit of synthesizing what we have witnessed and learned as participants in and observers of the COVID vaccination campaign. These are certainly not the only lessons or insights that matter, nor would they be the most important to some. They provide a summary of what we believe to be the fundamental issues that mattered most from our experience working with and supporting public health leaders throughout the COVID vaccination campaign. To reiterate, these five lessons are that

1. Funding matters;
2. Trust matters;
3. Local, national, and global action matters;
4. Nonpartisanship matters; and
5. Leadership matters.

Funding Matters

As we describe in our introduction to this book, America's governmental public health agencies entered the COVID pandemic underresourced and understaffed with portfolios of categorical work that limited their flexibility to respond to a novel health threat. Resources for vaccine administration were needed for several different COVID vaccination activities. These functions included expanding the vaccine administration workforce, hiring outreach and other community-based public health workers, staffing and equipping local and state operated vaccination sites to complement clinical and pharmacy locations, and expanding vaccine education and vaccine confidence. Also included, among many other functions, were purchasing supplies for clinical operations not otherwise covered and initiating data system modifications and updates to existing vaccine-tracking systems and immunization information systems, mortuary space, and hospital status-tracking systems.

And, as we described in Chapter 3, despite CDC director Dr. Robert Redfield's estimate that public health agencies would need between $5.5 billion to $6 billion to effectively support the COVID vaccine administration campaign, leaders of Operation Warp Speed and other Department of Health and Human Services officials did not see the need and overruled his professional judgment. In November 2020, public health agencies were planning for the largest vaccination campaign in US history to start in just four weeks with a budget of about $1 per American for the effort.

Ultimately, after significant advocacy by public health leaders and governors, Congress appropriated additional funding to support federal, state, and local vaccination activities and a host of other public health efforts. These resources allowed states to effectively roll out vaccines, but the battles over funding for COVID were reminiscent of earlier funding debates over how to sustain the capacity of governmental public health agencies to respond to other public health emergencies.

For many years, public health advocates and practitioners have called for sustained and increased federal investments in public health infrastructure to improve the capacity of the public health system to respond to everyday disease threats as well as public health emergencies. While the US Congress has always responded to funding requests for major public health disasters and events, including Zika, Ebola, H1N1, and the opioid overdose epidemic, these investments have often come in the midst of crises and have never been continued to support the kind of sustained capacity needed to build a local, state, and federal system capable of responding adequately to emerging disease threats on a continuous basis.

In a hearing held on March 10, 2022, by the House Homeland Security Subcommittee on Emergency Preparedness, Response, and Recovery, Mississippi's state health officer Dr. Thomas Dobbs stated:

> One of the challenges that we face is this funding up and down, where sometimes we will get specific money to address a specific issue like Zika, or like Ebola. But then, as that crisis resolves, or sort of diminishes, then we are—have to contract back to a state of acceptable, but not sufficient readiness . . . [W]e can't really make sure that we advance those efforts unless we have some steady funding, and don't go through this perpetual sort-of roller coaster cycle of funding for one thing that is limited to that, don't have the flexibility then to use it for the next thing.[14]

The roller coaster cycle of boom-bust,[15] or panic-neglect,[16] that has characterized public health emergency response has undermined readiness and kept state and territorial health agencies from building the sustained capacity to anticipate and rapidly respond to public health emergencies of any scale and consequence.

Fortunately, the boom-bust cycle of public health funding may soon be interrupted, at least for the near term, given the Biden administration's and some congressional support for core public health infrastructure. The CDC's recently announced $3.9 billion, five-year public health workforce and data modernization program will be a significant funding source for key public health activities at the state and local levels.[17] In addition, funded in the FFY22 federal budget was a new Public Health Infrastructure Fund that similarly provides flexible resources to states and territories and may serve as the long-term vehicle to fund state and territorial health agency infrastructure into the future. The $200 million appropriated for the fund in fiscal year 2022 may seem small compared to the emergency investments for public health that Congress made throughout COVID, but it is a start.[18]

Before COVID, experts estimated that an additional $4.5 billion was needed annually to support the foundational public health services all governmental agencies should provide to protect and promote health at the local and state levels.[19] Post-COVID estimates will certainly be higher, given the gaps and deficiencies identified through the pandemic. The overall economic losses of the COVID response in the United States are estimated to be almost $5 trillion, and globally approximately $16 trillion.[20] At a February 24, 2021, House Committee on Appropriations subcommittee hearing entitled "Ready or Not: US Public Health Infrastructure," US Congressman Tom Cole (R-OK) stated, "As I have told our own side and I think the last year has illustrated to all of us, sometimes you need to spend billions to save trillions and just look at the cost of what this pandemic has been,"[21] referring to the need to invest in governmental public health infrastructure before, not during, a pandemic to save trillions in economic losses that might result.

As Claire Hannan, MPH, told us in our March 17, 2022, oral interview with her, expecting a robust public health response without adequate funding to support it is like creating a "wishlist." The time to debate the need for adequately funding public health emergency response is not in the middle of one. If there are any positive outcomes associated with COVID, one may be that there is finally broad recognition of the vital work of governmental public health and the need to support and sustain the capacities built to respond to COVID to help improve the overall public health enterprise.

We still have a way to go to build a public health system that has enough steady state capacity to quickly respond to emerging health threats. But these new resources will help sustain and enhance future pandemic preparedness and should facilitate higher levels of routine vaccination in the future. In the final analysis, the key to ensuring high vaccine coverage is having a fully functioning immunization program for both children and adults before it is needed in an emergency. As one of the nation's foremost experts on immunization administration, Dr. Walter Orenstein told us the most important lesson from COVID is, in his view, that we need a fully funded and functioning adult immunization program infrastructure before the next emergency arrives (author oral interview with Walter A. Orenstein, MD, February 21, 2022).

Trust Matters

The issue of trust gets to the core of what drives vaccine confidence. As research presented in Chapter 6 has illustrated, societies with high trust in government and interpersonal trust had fewer COVID infections and higher COVID vaccination coverage than those with lower trust. In the United States, mistrust and distrust of government weakened public confidence in the safety of COVID vaccines.

Two major threads of distrust emerged during COVID. The first thread concerns lack of vaccine confidence in communities of color. Many studies have found that vaccine hesitancy is higher among Black and brown Americans as a consequence of their lived experience of racism and discrimination in the health care system. This includes a shared history of medical experimentation and abuses that have taken place from the very beginning of our country's founding. The second thread is rooted in distrust of public health authority as it is perceived to oppose personal liberty. With COVID, this thread also reflected a seemingly growing mistrust of science, the process by which vaccines are developed, and their safety is assured.

Building COVID vaccine confidence among people of color was a significant goal of governmental public health agencies. Engaging trusted members of different communities to share their support for vaccination with their family and social networks was a key trust building strategy, as was addressing vaccine complacency and convenience. Many local campaigns went out to neighborhoods, sometimes door to door or "phone to phone," to promote vaccination and build trust by sharing the benefits of COVID vaccines to both individuals and communities. The Biden administration and state and local public health agencies put equity front and center as a goal. Such efforts worked. The COVID vaccine hesitancy gap between Black and white Americans narrowed over time, and the percentage of Hispanic Americans and Native Alaskans/America Indians vaccinated is higher than the rate for white Americans relative to their percentage of the US population.[2]

The task now is to assess the various efforts of public health agencies to increase vaccine confidence among communities of color, with an eye toward sharing what made the public health agencies effective and how to best sustain them. Addressing structural racism in the health care and public health system is also a significant and urgent priority for many national public health organizations as we move into the future.[22,23]

Building trust in vaccines among Americans who question the science of their development, have doubts about their safety, or believe prevalent vaccine mis- and disinformation remains a persistent challenge. Unfortunately, the extreme politicization of COVID vaccines coupled with the distrust many Americans have in government appears to be having a spillover effect and may be further reducing routine vaccination rates for children and adults.

A two-pronged strategy is needed. The first approach, similar to building confidence in communities of color, should be to maximize the vaccine confidence messages delivered by trusted messengers. The research by de Beaumont and Frank Luntz reviewed in Chapter 6, as well as the many earlier studies of vaccine hesitancy, provides a helpful place to start in redoubling our efforts.

The second prong of the strategy needs to be holding social media platforms and their content creators accountable for spreading false or misleading information that is contributing to mistrust and distrust of vaccines. We further recognize that both Facebook and Twitter have policies in place that ban sharing deliberate misinformation about COVID vaccines. But more is needed: a March 2022 study found that in the case of Facebook, the impact of the ban has been modest.[24]

Because it is extremely difficult for public health agencies to counter the sheer volume of online anti-vaccination content and anti-science conspiracies, something must be done on a massive scale to reel in the myths and falsehoods these channels allow to circulate. Until then, public health is fighting a losing battle to counter online disinformation about vaccine science.

Humility plays a significant role in building authentic and empathetic trust-based relationships. The ability to say "I was wrong," or "I don't know" goes a long way in establishing the vulnerability individuals need to trust one another. Unfortunately, hubris was far more common during the COVID pandemic than humility. In efforts to portray confidence and reassurance, many public officials got the initial facts wrong and had to backtrack on public statements or dug in on positions that were no longer true based on new data. Hubris eroded trust by conveying certainty despite the incredible uncertainty associated with a previously unknown and constantly evolving virus.

Dr. Anthony Fauci, one of the most visible experts in the COVID response, stressed the importance of humility in his practice of medicine and in his leadership. Often cited as one of the most trustworthy spokespersons over the course of the pandemic, at a March 2021 virtual forum sponsored by the University of Chicago, he stated:

> You should be flexible enough and humble enough to know that, in fact, you've got to go with the data that you have—and if that means changing something that you said, you should not feel badly or even guilty about having to do that . . . I get more humble as the years go by because I realize how much I don't know.[25]

As great as our scientific advances have been, there is still much we do not know about the COVID virus. We are watching science evolve and knowledge expand in real time. This means recommendations and guidelines will change based on new evidence. There is humility in recognizing that changes were frustrating to the public and that any changes must be communicated as clearly as possible in the future.

Humility also means that strategies must be adaptable on the basis of facts on the ground. For example, hopes of achieving herd immunity through the vaccination campaign were largely dashed when it became clear that the virus was mutating rapidly and that available vaccines had waning immunity requiring new boosters and potentially new formulations. Asked about how herd immunity as a strategy has evolved, Dr. Aisha Jha, who later became the White House COVID response coordinator, told listeners to a February 2022 ASTHO *Public Health Review Morning Edition* podcast:

> I think we've all had to do a mental kind of update on what we think about what we mean by herd immunity. At this point in the United States, I'm guessing 90, 93% of Americans have some immunity against this virus, either from a prior infection or from vaccines. And yet, we saw Omicron's surge kind of rip across the nation with impunity. And so, that means the idea that we're going to have herd immunity, and that's going to wipe the virus out or kind of suppress it for a long time, is wishful thinking because you have waning immunity,

you have a highly contagious virus that can break through immunity, at least in terms of causing infection. And so, I don't see herd immunity as a strategy.[26]

A crucial lesson from the vaccine campaign was that public health and health care professionals were not just delivering vaccine, they were delivering on trust. This campaign was not just a technical and scientific challenge, but it was also an emotional and relational one.

Future efforts to respond to public health emergencies must consider both the necessary technical requirements of such a response and also the social, emotional, and attitudinal factors that will promote or inhibit individual and community health behaviors. This lesson was learned far too late in the response to COVID, and health officials have been playing catch-up ever since.

Local, National, and Global Action Matters

A maxim of disaster management is "All disasters are local." Emergencies play out most clearly at the local level, and local capacity is critical to emergency preparedness and response. Indeed, COVID started as a local emergency with reports of a cluster of pneumonia of unknown cause in Wuhan City, Hubei Province, China, in December 2019. As the new virus quickly spread, the emergency grew in scale and scope, becoming a public health emergency of international concern just weeks later on January 30, 2020.

One of the major lessons from the COVID vaccination campaign is that the work of turning vaccines into vaccinations takes place at the local, and even hyperlocal, level. Vaccination efforts were carried out block by block and neighborhood by neighborhood in many places to make it as convenient as possible to get vaccinated. Mobile vans and traveling public health nurses extended vaccine clinics from hospitals, health centers, clinics, and pharmacies into hard-to-reach areas and communities too small to support a brick-and-mortar health facility. Planes delivered vaccine to remote villages in Alaska, as well as to island states and territories in the Atlantic and Pacific not connected by roads or rails.

Getting vaccine to every community in America was a national effort, but the on-the-ground reality of administering vaccine in every city and town in the country varied locally depending on existing infrastructure, geography, and politics. State and local health departments and their private-sector partners had to coordinate the thousand details that presented themselves at the start of the vaccination campaign another thousand times over in communities across the country.

While standard planning assumptions and centralized guidance helped steer vaccine distribution and administration, no one-size-fits-all plan would ever work for every community in America. Instead, state, territorial, and local health officers adapted, tailored, cut, and replaced guidance documents issued nationally to make them fit local conditions and address local needs. The reality of state variation and the diversity of local implementation strategies is why it is so critical that national public health response efforts, led federally from Washington, DC, or Atlanta, have an explicit and intentional process to dialogue with and learn from state and local public health leaders across the country in real time.

So many opportunities to gather ground truth and consider the many ways that decisions have unintended consequences at the local level were missed in the planning of the national vaccination campaign. Throughout the COVID response, state and local partners consistently requested routine, deliberate, and predecisional engagement from federal partners. These engagement opportunities were often ad hoc and limited, delayed, or declined. Federal officials in both administrations often told state and local partners what they needed without ever asking first. Federal officials in both administrations have withheld upcoming policy changes that significantly affect state and local public health response efforts because they wanted to get information to the media first and feared leaks.

Future public health responses must include early and intentional engagement of governmental public health partners in a structured and systematic manner to avoid repeating many of the same implementation missteps and misunderstandings that arose throughout the vaccine distribution and administration campaign. This will require humility and trust.

Juxtaposed against the hyperlocal reality of COVID vaccination planning is the global spread and scale of COVID worldwide. While America's vaccine nationalism gave way to vaccine diplomacy in the spring of 2021, global efforts to vaccinate low-resource countries continue to suffer from limited investments from donor nations. This should concern us all, as preventing COVID in the future means addressing the pandemic worldwide. If the virus mutates and spreads, it remains a threat to all of us. As Dr. Tom Frieden reminds us in Chapter 7, "A virus anywhere is just a plane ride away."[27]

The term *glocal*, meaning "reflecting or characterized by both local and global considerations,"[28] may be most apt in describing where we find ourselves today with COVID response. The last mile of vaccination administration happens at the hyperlocal level, but the global challenge to the world's health presented by COVID and the need for an international response make it a global concern as well. As we plan for future pandemics, including the emergent monkeypox outbreak now spreading worldwide, it would behoove us to take such a *glocal* perspective by recognizing both the need for local response and the need for global intervention to stop the disease transmission.

Nonpartisanship Matters

COVID emerged in the United States amid incredible political divisiveness and partisanship. To paraphrase former White House COVID Task Force coordinator Dr. Birx, a presidential election year is a terrible, and dangerous, time to have a pandemic.[29]

From the beginning of COVID, it appeared the Trump administration's major concern was not the public's health but how to keep the American economy growing at its bullish rate even with the rise of a highly transmissible and potentially deadly new virus. Sustaining economic growth and a booming stock market were viewed by the president's team as critical to winning his reelection bid. As a result, President Trump and his surrogates downplayed the severity of the virus and were initially extremely wary of taking any action that might result in an economic slowdown.[30,31,32]

The pandemic soon became a partisan minefield with Republicans criticizing efforts by public health authorities to contain and mitigate the virus. Democrats were seen as overstating the threat of COVID in a bid to make the president look bad and lose momentum in the contentious campaign season. Disagreements between Democratic governors and the White House about what resources they needed to stop the spread of COVID became public spectacles and sideshows, especially in President Trump's rows with Governors Gretchen Whitmer of Michigan and Andrew Cuomo of New York.[33,34] Many Republicans loyal to the president pushed back on mask mandates, gathering restrictions, and business closures as government overreach and overreaction. Plans to expand voting by mail or increase drive-thru ballot drop-off sites so that individuals could vote without potential exposure to COVID were viewed as Democratic ploys to promote voter fraud.

COVID vaccines became a flashpoint for both sides. President Trump wanted to tout successful vaccine development as a highlight of his first term but at the same time downplayed the need for vaccines by minimizing the severity of COVID. The vaccine review process undertaken by the Food and Drug Administration (FDA) became symbolic of the fight: the president believed review and approval was being deliberately slowed until after the election, whereas the Biden–Harris team was skeptical of the process and its speed. Pfizer announced its vaccine efficacy studies on November 9, 2020, just six days after the November 3 election, raising Trump's ire and fueling suspicions of a Democratic-FDA-Pfizer conspiracy against him.

Ultimately, neither side was right, according to Kathrin Jansen, Pfizer's head of research and development. In an interview with *ScienceInsider*, she told reporter Jon Cohen:

> Quite frankly, we had no time and still have no time to deal with politics. We are at this 24/7, thousands of people working diligently to make this work. And for us, it was never about politics, it was always about just the disaster that we were in the middle of, all of us globally, seeing the devastation and the deaths.[35]

But the partisan battling over vaccine development cast a lasting shadow over its ultimate administration.

For the first time that we are aware of in our history, the use of a safe, effective, FDA-authorized product split significantly along partisan lines, with Republicans considerably less likely to be vaccinated than Democrats. You would never expect to see partisan differences in the use of other lifesaving interventions like angioplasty or chemotherapy, so to many of us it is baffling to see the split with COVID vaccine. But as Claire Hannan, MPH, shared with us in our March 17, 2022, oral interview, "I think the unfortunate thing is that people are using vaccination to make a political statement."

Although public health has always been political, however, it has not always been so bitterly partisan. Dr. Tom Frieden told National Public Radio in July 2021:

> There's no doubt that politics plays a major role in public health decisions. You sometimes hear people say, let's get the politics out of public health. Well, public health is the activity of communities getting safer and healthier. And there are many political decisions that happen during that process. What's problematic is when partisanship gets in the way because there really shouldn't be a Democratic or Republican way to control pandemics. There should be a scientific way, or a way that ignores the science, and let's choose the scientific way.[36]

Before the onslaught of COVID, there had been general agreement that regardless of political party, following the science to stem the spread of disease was a good thing. But throughout the pandemic, public health measures were politicized and, as we saw in Chapter 6, led to heightened vaccine hesitancy and support for anti-science beliefs among Republicans in particular.

Former secretary of the Kansas Department of Health and Environment Dr. Lee Norman was one of several health officials subject to death threats in his state because of mask mandates, business closures, and vaccine recommendations. Shortly after his resignation in November 2021, Rachel Maddow interviewed him on the *Rachel Maddow Show* about the impact of extreme partisanship. He told her:

> I think the hardest thing, particularly in a state like Kansas, many other states where there's such bitter partisanship, and especially in a state like Kansas where the governor is one party and both houses of the legislature are the other side, then it really gets partisan, and I think what gets lost in this is the fact that we should put people's health first, and I think a lot of times partisanship is trumping public health, and it should be absolutely the other way around.[37]

Dr. Anthony Fauci, himself the target of threats that required him to have the protection of a security detail, had warned of the dangers of partisanship a year earlier when he urged Americans to move beyond the partisan divide inflaming the COVID crisis. In a November 2020 interview with *USA Today*, he said:

> We've got to say, "OK, folks, enough is enough with this political divisiveness, with this claiming that people are making things up. Get rid of these ridiculous conspiracy theories and realize this is a public health crisis." This is real, and if the divisiveness is so severe that

people don't think it's real when people are flooding hospitals and dying at a rate that we haven't seen with a disease of this type in 102 years, I hope that's enough of a stimulus for us to drop back as a nation and say, "Hey, folks, we got to start talking to each other about what this divide is between us."[38]

The danger of partisanship is that it puts political agendas first, not people's health. As we learned, thousands of Americans died as a result. We should all heed the advice shared by Dr. Fauci and "start talking to each other" about the divide between us. If political posturing and partisan competition can so significantly erode trust in science and our trust in each other, those conversations must start now. Former defense secretary Mark Esper reflects on the accomplishments of Operation Warp Speed and the hope it brought at a difficult time in history, suggesting the effort could be a starting place for unity in post-pandemic America:

Despite all the politics of the moment, I am confident that historians will look back upon [Operation Warp Speed] as the incredible partnership and accomplishment that it was. Not only did it deliver hope to the American people when they needed it most, it delivered on its promise to create a vaccine by the end of the year. With well over five hundred thousand dead to COVID-19, our economy in a poor state, and the social fabric of the country in tatters, a safe and effective vaccine was always going to be our best bet for a return to normal, whatever that will look like in a postpandemic world.[39(p291)]

Dr. Kelly Moore, former immunization program manager for the State of Tennessee, stated the danger of "us" versus "them" thinking, telling us:

We needed everybody to really be on board with supporting and encouraging the vaccines and championing them and celebrating them. And having a unified voice that wherever people looked it isn't about just having one or two champions or experts saying this is the right thing, but everybody consistently being supportive, and not in a way that whitewashes challenges . . . And instead we found a politicized process somehow, and it became an us and them thing. And we never overcame that. And now we have people who would rather die than submit to a vaccine. I sometimes paraphrase Freud and say, "Sometimes a vaccine is just a vaccine." (author oral interview with Kelly Moore, MD, MPH, February 25, 2022)

Leadership Matters

At a May 2022 closed-door summit hosted by ASTHO and the CDC Foundation, the nation's health officers met with key federal officials to discuss plans to respond to potential COVID surges in the summer and fall. While the meeting was ostensibly called to get ahead of the next COVID surge, something very different was the result: state and federal health officials began to share the personal toll of leading during a pandemic. The burden of their responsibilities in leading teams of thousands of public health professionals through a global pandemic came through loud and clear.

Leadership matters. Without it, organizations can become listless, be ossified, and fail to evolve. No major undertaking can be carried out without it. COVID leadership required a tremendous amount of energy from leaders who had to lead through uncertainty and cope with tremendous adversity while experiencing COVID both personally and professionally. Many state and local health leaders became public health celebrities in their jurisdictions with Facebook fan club pages and with T-shirts, bobble heads, votive candles, and even candy bars with their likeness widely shared throughout their states. Many state health officers unfortunately also became targets of hate and harassment.

The Honorable Mike Leavitt, former governor of Utah and secretary of the Department of Health and Human services during the George W. Bush administration, presciently stated, "In advance of a pandemic, anything you say sounds alarmist. After a pandemic starts, everything you've done is inadequate."[40] In Secretary Leavitt's case, the threat was bird flu, not coronavirus, but the statement rings very true to the dilemma faced by so many who led through COVID.

In our view, leadership is the act of setting a vision, bringing people together around a common goal, achieving clarity of purpose, and motivating others to achieve it. In the vaccination campaign, there are incredible examples of leaders across the country and around the globe doing just that. Operation Warp Speed leaders had vision, clarity of purpose, and execution: their goal was clear, the troops were motivated. Their success, along with the leadership of thousands of public health professionals at the state and local levels, should be celebrated.

Of course, there are also plentiful examples of poor leadership throughout COVID. We have highlighted several of those in earlier chapters, not to add to the chorus of criticism many of these individuals face but to demonstrate that bad leadership, or lack of leadership, has a tremendous cost. The costs include missed opportunities, confusion, communication delays, and wasted effort—and most important, needless illness and preventable death.

THE STRUGGLE OF SUCCESS

These foregoing five lessons are not the only ones we have learned, but they certainly encompass the major themes we have gathered from our interviews, observations, and participation in the public health response to COVID. To complement these lessons and learn more, we believe a national effort needs to be initiated now to review, document, synthesize, and share other insights from the field in this response. The danger in not learning from history is repeating it. And we can guarantee that repeating the experience of COVID is something every public health professional wants to avoid.

From our point of view, public health and its many partners should be lauded for their work to successfully vaccinate America. We also acknowledge, however, that it is difficult to fully celebrate the success of the vaccination campaign considering two important points. First, a significant percentage of the US population continue to lack confidence in COVID vaccination, minimize the need to be vaccinated, and are either delaying or refusing to get vaccinated. While achieving 100% vaccination of all eligible adults was never a realistic goal, opportunities exist even now to push the COVID vaccination rate in America higher. Celebrating success does not mean we are done with the effort, but it does mean pausing to observe just how far we have come. This achievement is even more amazing given the vilification of public health activities and tremendous pushback to vaccination efforts from many Americans, some of whom may never be vaccinated.

Second, we must recognize, with a great deal of humility and sadness, that over one million Americans have died from COVID-related illness. If one measures the success of governmental public health work in its purest form as the prevention of avoidable morbidity and mortality, we have much more cause for mourning than we do for celebration. We certainly understand this point and do not seek to minimize a death toll that is far too high. In a searing essay, *Atlantic* writer Ed Yong reflected on the immense grief caused by the now more than one million COVID deaths. "That number—the sum total of a million individual tragedies," he wrote, "is almost too large to grasp, and only a few professions have borne visceral witness to the pandemic's immense scale."[41]

Imagine how that grief is compounded in those whose profession is to promote and administer the single simple and effective intervention that can prevent serious illness and death but cannot effectively reach all who could benefit. If we can somehow channel this grief into effective action, we believe it can be the impetus for an even harder push to finish the job of fully vaccinating as many Americans as possible in the future.

The COVID vaccination story is one that affects everyone on the planet. We also acknowledge that no one knows exactly how this story ends. While the push to increase vaccine booster rates and new, expanded vaccine eligibility of children age six months to five years has broadened the vaccination effort, we continue to see little increase in demand for vaccines nationwide. Likewise, COVAX has reported that demand for COVID vaccines has similarly softened worldwide.[42]

New bivalent vaccines to target COVID variants became available in early fall 2022, but it remains an open question as to how many will seek those out, given the overwhelming desire of so many to just "move on" from COVID. We too want to move on from COVID. Moving on does not mean ignoring the lessons of the past two and a half years, however, or failing to recognize the Herculean effort it took to turn vaccines into vaccinations. Instead, moving on means admitting the agonizing truth about what happens when an unknown virus emerges amid extreme partisan divisiveness and presents itself to an underresourced public health system—and it means learning from the experience.

Moving on also means honoring the work of so many committed and talented public health and health care professionals who carried out the historic and successful race to vaccinate America. It certainly was not seamless, but the race to administer over 600 million doses over the past 18 months and save over two million lives is historic and unprecedented. It deserves to be celebrated. Kelly Moore, MD, MPH, echoed this point in our February 25, 2022, oral interview, adding, "They deserve to be celebrated, and next time they deserve to be listened to as well." We hope the accomplishment of such a historic achievement also provides the motivation not to give up until the job is done.

REFERENCES

1. Barry JM. *The Great Influenza: The Epic Story of the Deadliest Plague in History*. London, England: Penguin Books; 2009.

2. Centers for Disease Control and Prevention. CDC COVID data tracker. Available at: https://covid.cdc.gov/covid-data-tracker/#vaccinations_vacc-people-additional-dose-totalpop. Accessed September 24, 2022.

3. Ndugga N, Hill L, Artiga S, Haldar S. Latest data on COVID-19 vaccinations by race/ethnicity. Kaiser Family Foundation. July 14, 2022. Available at: https://www.kff.org/coronavirus-covid-19/issue-brief/latest-data-on-covid-19-vaccinations-by-race-ethnicity. Accessed September 20, 2022.

4. CNBC. We need to put more resources in place for vaccine distribution: expert [Dr. Marcus Plescia]. December 1, 2020. Available at: https://www.cnbc.com/video/2020/12/01/we-need-to-put-more-resources-in-place-for-vaccine-distribution-expert.html?&qsearchterm=marcus+plescia. Accessed September 20, 2022.

5. Bryant-Genevier J, Rao C, Lopes-Cardozo B, et al. Symptoms of depression, anxiety, post-traumatic stress disorder, and suicidal ideation among state, tribal, local, and territorial public health workers during the COVID-19 pandemic—United States, March–April 2021. *MMWR*. 2021;70(48):1680–1685.

6. Association of State and Territorial Health Officials. Public Health Review Morning Edition. Episode 122: ASTHO's new resiliency program. February 18, 2022. Available at: https://newscast.astho.org/122-asthos-new-resiliency-program. Accessed September 24, 2022.

7. Health Resources & Services Administration. Health and Public Safety Workforce Resiliency Technical Assistance Center (HPSWRTAC). HRSA-22-111. Available at: https://www.hrsa.gov/grants/find-funding/hrsa-22-111. Accessed September 20, 2022.

8. Schneider E, Shah A, Sah P, et al. Impact of US COVID-19 vaccination efforts: an update on averted deaths, hospitalizations, and health care costs through March 2022. Commonwealth Fund. April 8, 2022. Available at: https://www.commonwealthfund.org/blog/2022/impact-us-covid-19-vaccination-efforts-march-update. Accessed September 20, 2022.

9. Congressional Research Service. The US government's role in domestic and global COVID-19 vaccine supply and distribution: frequently asked questions. February 17, 2022. Available at: https://www.everycrsreport.com/reports/IF12013.html. Accessed September 20, 2022.

10. Briand S. It is impossible to predict the evolution of the COVID-19 pandemic. LinkedIn. February 6, 2022. Available at: https://www.linkedin.com/posts/sylvie-briand-20a9bb15_covid-globalhealth-pandemicresponse-activity-6896119756747874304-D1r-?. Accessed September 24, 2022.

11. Davis R. Opinion: visit to historic cemetery shows power of vaccinations. *Atlanta Journal-Constitution*. October 30, 2021. Available at: https://www.ajc.com/opinion/opinion-visit-to-historic-cemetery-shows-power-of-vaccinations/VGZMNQOI3ZDZBE6AN4LMM7CAJY. Accessed September 20, 2022.

12. Thornton C, Fernando C. World Health Organization chief says monkeypox is now a global emergency. *USA Today*. July 23, 2022. Updated July 24, 2022. Available at: https://www.usatoday.com/story/news/health/2022/07/23/who-monkeypox-outbreak-global-emergency/10134299002. Accessed September 24, 2022.

13. Diamond D. Monkeypox is "a public health emergency," US health secretary declares. *Washington Post*. Updated August 4, 2022. Available at: Available at: https://www.washingtonpost.com/health/2022/08/04/monkeypox-public-health-emergency-united-states-becerra. Accessed September 20, 2022.

14. US House Committee on Homeland Security, Subcommittee on Emergency Preparedness, Response, and Recovery. Community perspectives on coronavirus preparedness and response. [Hearing transcript]. US Government Publishing Office. March 10, 2010. Available at: https://www.govinfo.gov/content/pkg/CHRG-116hhrg42343/html/CHRG-116hhrg42343.htm. Accessed September 24, 2022.

15. Trust for America's Health. The impact of chronic underfunding on America's public health system: trends, risks, and recommendations, 2021. May 2021. Available at: https://www.tfah.org/wp-content/uploads/2021/05/2021_PHFunding_Fnl.pdf. Accessed September 20, 2022.

16. Yong E. America is zooming through the pandemic panic-neglect cycle. *Atlantic*. March 17, 2022. Available at: https://www.theatlantic.com/health/archive/2022/03/congress-covid-spending-bill/627090. Accessed September 20, 2022.

17. Centers for Disease Control and Prevention. Center for Surveillance, Epidemiology, and Laboratory Services. OE22-2203 strengthening US public health infrastructure, workforce, and data systems. Summer 2022. Available at: https://www.cdc.gov/workforce/resources/infrastructuregrant/pdfs/PHI_Grant_One_Pager.pdf. Accessed September 20, 2022.

18. Consolidated Appropriations Act of 2022, HR 2471, 117th Cong (2022). Available at: https://www.congress.gov/bill/117th-congress/house-bill/2471/text. Accessed September 20, 2022.

19. Hines M. Bipartisan leaders call for $4.5B for public health infrastructure. *RESOLVE*. March 17, 2020. Available at: https://www.resolve.ngo/blog/Bipartisan-Leaders-Call-for-45B-for-Public-Health-Infrastructure.htm. Accessed September 20, 2022.

20. Cutler DM, Summers LH. The COVID-19 pandemic and the $16 trillion virus. *JAMA*. 2020;324(15):1495–1496. doi:10.1001/jama.2020.19759.

21. House Committee on Appropriations. Hearing: labor, health and human services, education, and related agencies. Ready or not: US public health infrastructure. February 24, 2021. Available at: https://appropriations.house.gov/subcommittees/labor-health-and-human-services-education-and-related-agencies-117th-congress/congress_hearing?page=1. Accessed September 24, 2022.

22. Association of State and Territorial Health Officials. Achieving optimal health for all by eliminating structural racism. 2021. Available at: https://www.astho.org/globalassets/pdf/policy-statements/achieving-optimal-health-for-all-eliminating-structural-racism.pdf. Accessed September 20, 2022.

23. American Public Health Association. Structural racism is a public health crisis: impact on the Black community. APHA LB20-04. October 24, 2020. Available at: https://www.apha.org/policies-and-advocacy/public-health-policy-statements/policy-database/2021/01/13/structural-racism-is-a-public-health-crisis. Accessed September 20, 2022.

24. Gu J, Dor A, Li K, et al. The impact of Facebook's vaccine misinformation policy on user endorsements of vaccine content: an interrupted time series analysis. *Vaccine.* 2022;40(14):2209–2214. doi:10.1016/j.vaccine.2022.02.062.

25. Wang J. For Dr. Fauci, COVID-19 has underscored value of humility in public policy. University of Chicago Harris School of Public Policy. March 5, 2021. Available at: https://harris.uchicago.edu/news-events/news/dr-fauci-covid-19-has-underscored-value-humility-public-policy. Accessed September 20, 2022.

26. Association of State and Territorial Health Officials. Is COVID-19 in Retreat? Transcript. *Public Health Review Morning Edition.* February 15, 2022. Accessed August 14, 2022. https://newscast.astho.org/119-is-covid-19-in-retreat/#transcript. Accessed August 14, 2022.

27. Overman S. CDC director catalogs health threats that are 'just a plane ride away." National Press Club. Available at: https://www.press.org/newsroom/cdc-director-catalogs-health-threats-are-just-plane-ride-away. Accessed September 24, 2022.

28. Dictionary.com. Glocal. Available at: https://www.dictionary.com/browse/glocal. Accessed August 14, 2022.

29. CBS News. Transcript: Dr. Deborah Birx on "Face the Nation," January 24, 2021. January 24, 2021. Available at: https://www.cbsnews.com/news/transcript-deborah-birx-on-face-the-nation-january-24-2021. Accessed September 24 2022.

30. Woodward B. *Rage.* London, England: Simon & Schuster; 2020.

31. Slavitt A. *Preventable: The Inside Story of How Leadership Failures, Politics, and Selfishness Doomed the US Coronavirus Response.* New York, NY: St. Martin's Press; 2021.

32. Birx DL. *Silent Invasion: The Untold Story of the Trump Administration, Covid-19, and Preventing the Next Pandemic before It's Too Late.* New York, NY: Harper, an imprint of HarperCollins Publishers; 2022.

33. Bradner E. "That governor is me": Gretchen Whitmer takes on Trump as coronavirus cases rise in Michigan. *CNN.* March 30, 2020. Available at: https://www.cnn.com/2020/03/29/politics/gretchen-whitmer-donald-trump-coronavirus/index.html. Accessed September 20, 2022.

34. Forgey Q, Choi M. Trump downplays need for ventilators as New York begs to differ. *Politico.* March 27, 2020. Available at: https://www.politico.com/news/2020/03/26/trump-ventilators-coronavirus-151311. Accessed September, 2022.

35. Cohen J. Fact check: no evidence supports Trump's claim that COVID-19 vaccine result was suppressed to sway election. *Science.* November 11, 2020. Available at: https://www.science.org/content/article/fact-check-no-evidence-supports-trump-s-claim-covid-19-vaccine-result-was-suppressed. Accessed September 20, 2022.

36. Former CDC director discusses balancing science and politics in pandemic response. *Weekend Edition Saturday.* National Public Radio. July 31, 2021. Available at: https://www .npr.org/2021/07/31/1023146072/former-cdc-director-discusses-balancing-science-and-politics-in-pandemic-response. Accessed September 20, 2022.

37. MSNBC. Transcript: The Rachel Maddow Show, 12/8/21. December 8, 2021. Available at: https://www.msnbc.com/transcripts/transcript-rachel-maddow-show-12-8-21-n1285857. Accessed September 20, 2022.

38. Carroll N. Backstory: Anthony Fauci has had it with people who think COVID-19 is no worse than the flu. *USA Today.* November 20, 2020. Available at: https://www.usatoday.com/story/opinion/2020/11/20/anthony-fauci-covid-us-must-accept-how-dangerous-coronavirus-is-react/3778241001. Accessed September 20, 2022.

39. Esper, Mark. *A Sacred Oath: Memoirs of a Secretary of Defense during Extraordinary Times.* New York: William Morrow; 2022.

40. Avian Flu Diary, Quotable Quotes. May 17, 2007. Available at: https://afludiary.blogspot .com/2007/05/quotable-quotes.html. Accessed September 20, 2022.

41. Yong E. The final pandemic betrayal. *Atlantic.* May 25, 2022. Available at: https://www .theatlantic.com/health/archive/2022/04/us-1-million-covid-death-rate-grief/629537. Accessed September 24, 2022.

42. Ravelo JL. COVID-19 vaccine delivery and demand "slowing down." *Devex.* May 6, 2022. Available at: https://www.devex.com/news/covid-19-vaccine-delivery-and-demand-slowing-down-103187. Accessed September 24, 2022.

About the Authors

Dr. Michael Fraser serves as the Chief Executive Officer of the Association of State and Territorial Health Officials (ASTHO). Dr. Fraser is a dynamic leader in the health care and public health fields and has experience leading public health associations, medical societies, and the federal government. He has been featured in interviews with the *Washington Post, New York Times, The Wall Street Journal, Politico, The Hill*, CNN, Bloomberg, MSNBC, and other national and regional media outlets. Dr. Fraser is a coeditor and author of *A Public Health Guide to Ending the Opioid Crisis* with Jay Butler and coauthor of *A Communications Playbook for Public Officials: How to Effectively Manage the Message, the Media, and Yourself* with Robert Johnson. He is coeditor and author of the forthcoming *Handbook of Strategic Skills for Public Health Practice* with Brian Castrucci and author of the forthcoming *Leading Systems Change in Public Health: A Field Guide for Practitioners*. Dr. Fraser is an affiliated faculty in the Departments of Global and Community Health and Health Administration and Policy at the George Mason University, College of Health and Human Services. Prior to joining ASTHO, he served as the executive vice president and CEO of the Pennsylvania Medical Society. He served as CEO of the Association of Maternal and Child Health Programs (AMCHP) from 2007 to 2013.

Brent Ewig is a leader and advocate for public health. For close to three decades, he has worked with government agencies, nonprofit associations, foundations, and other interest groups in the global, federal, state, and local health policy arenas. He became Chief Policy and Government Relations Officer for the Association of Immunization Managers (AIM) in August 2022. He previously worked as a consultant policy advisor to AIM and Director of Policy and Government Affairs at the Association of Maternal and Child Health Programs (AMCHP). He also worked eight years at the Association of State and Territorial Health Officials (ASTHO), where he served as Principal Director for Prevention and Public Health.

Index

C